VOICES
OF CLASSICAL PILATES II

• Men's Work •

COLLECTED ESSAYS AND DIALOGUES

30 Classical Pilates Teachers & Students Share Their Lives and Work

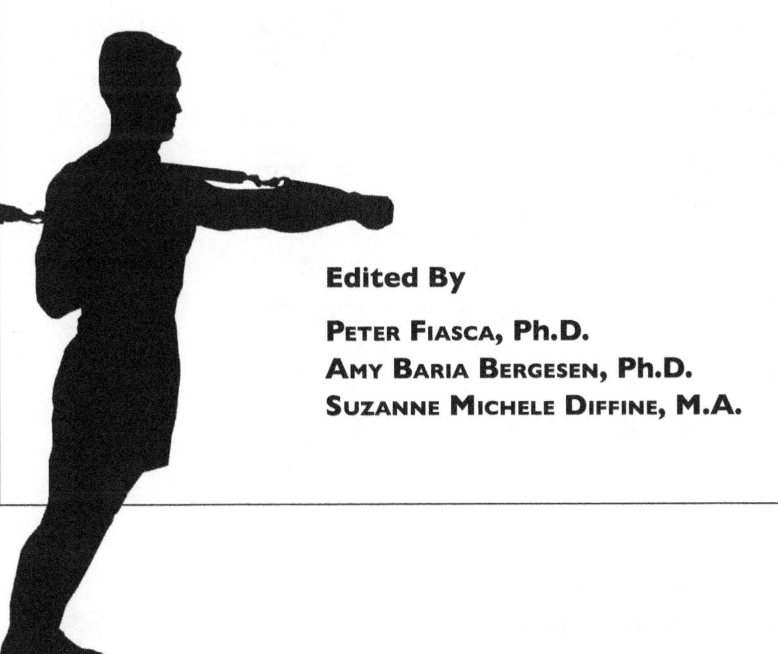

Edited By

PETER FIASCA, Ph.D.
AMY BARIA BERGESEN, Ph.D.
SUZANNE MICHELE DIFFINE, M.A.

Copyright © 2017 by PETER FIASCA.

All rights reserved under International and Pan-American Copyright Conventions. No part of this publication may be reproduced, stored in a retrieval system, or transmitted in any form or by any means, electronic, mechanical, photocopying, recording, or otherwise, without the prior written permission of the publisher. For information, contact Peter Fiasca via ClassicalPilates.net or telephone 215.205.8004.

First American Edition 2017

Voices of Classical Pilates II: Men's Work can be purchased through: ClassicalPilates.net

Library of Congress Control Number: 2017903531

ISBN: 978-0-9893693-3-6

Cover Art & Interior Layout: Joanna Libonati

Caution:

This book is not intended for treatment of any injuries.
Do not use as a replacement for medical care.
Obtain a physician's advice before starting any physical fitness program.

Table of Contents

(cont.)

Table of Contents (cont.)

Dedication

This book is dedicated to Joseph and Clara Pilates, as well as to my primary teachers, Romana Kryzanowska and Jay Grimes, who have preserved the full spectrum of Contrology with love, wisdom, and a wonderful sense of humor. It is equally important to acknowledge all the loyal, exceptionally skilled professionals who share their knowledge of Joseph Pilates' Traditional Method with students and future generations of faithful instructors.

-PETER FIASCA

Foreword

by

Peter Fiasca, Ph.D.

Amy Baria Bergesen, Ph.D.   Suzanne Michele Diffine, M.A.

With great pleasure, we present *Voices of Classical Pilates II: Men's Work.* We hope you enjoy this wonderful collection of essays and dialogues, focusing upon the work of men in Traditional Pilates technique. The lives and ideas of these 30 well-respected, professional Classical Pilates teachers and their hard-working students are truly fascinating and invigorating.

Voices of Classical Pilates II: Men's Work was over three years in the making, like our first collection of essays, *Voices of Classical Pilates*. This comprehensive collection of essays serves three important purposes: (1) to help preserve Joseph Pilates' Classical Method of mental and physical conditioning by focusing upon men's work; (2) to present a dynamic exchange of ideas and life experiences between individuals devoted to Classical Pilates; (3) to educate the public, as well as various professionals, about divergent perspectives within the value system of Traditional Pilates technique.

In *Voices of Classical Pilates: Men's Work* you will find these subjects and many more:

- Championship Football and Pilates
- An Olympic Athlete's Guidance
- A Cardiac Surgeon's Viewpoint
- Chiropractics and Contrology
- Men & The Powerhouse
- Gender Imbalance in Pilates
- Connecting Brain and Body
- Martial Arts & Classical Pilates
- International Perspectives
- Starting Pilates Over Age 50
- Teaching Men the Traditional Work
- Rehabilitation from a Sports Injury
- Men's Misperceptions of The Work
- Athletics & The Role of Pilates

The process of combining these powerful life experiences of strong male students and their seasoned, professional teachers has been deeply rewarding because their work has the potential to benefit everyone. We sincerely hope that *Voices of Classical Pilates II: Men's Work* helps bring you to a deeper—even more positive—connection with Traditional Pilates technique as well as with your life and professional work.

Chapter I

Pilates and Discovery

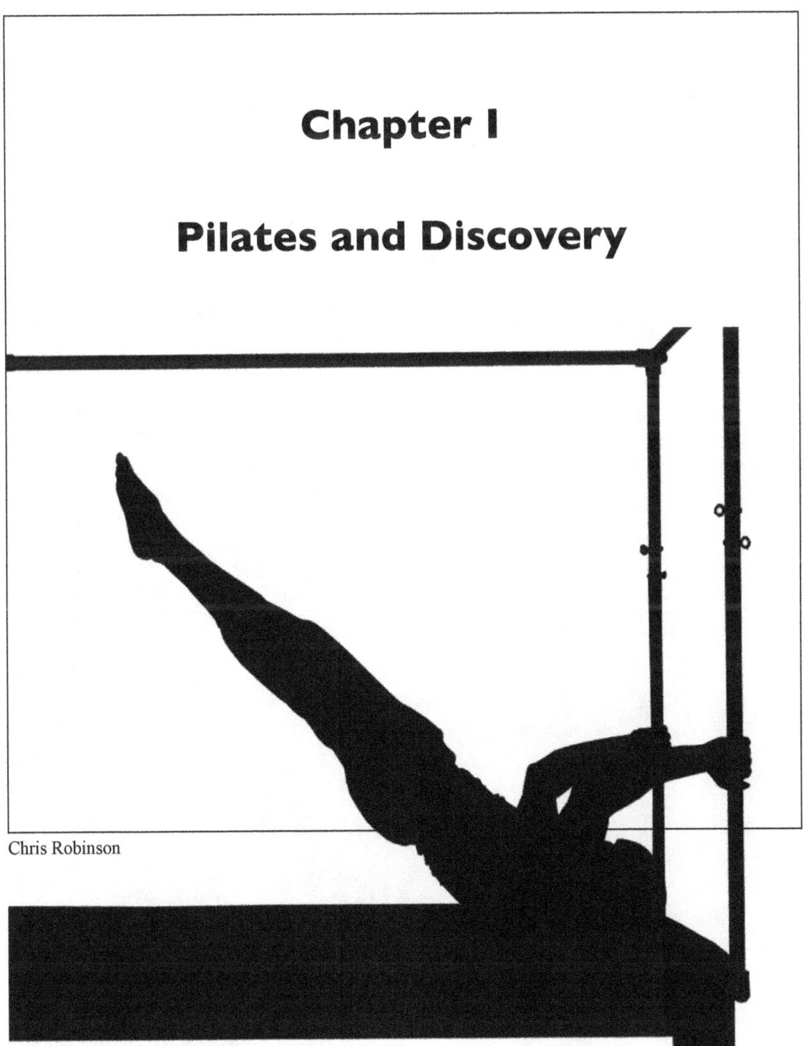

Chris Robinson

An Open Letter to Pilates Instructors

By Jay Grimes

Change comes through movement, not talking...

Dear Pilates Teacher,

You talk too much!

Have you ever had a client, perhaps for several years, who is dedicated and smart and who one day has a eureka moment and tells you something you have been telling them hundreds of times? Well guess what—you've been talking too much. Either the client has simply turned you off and doesn't listen, or they have understood mentally but were not ready to understand physically.

You actually cannot teach Pilates. Pilates comes from within. People have to discover it in their own body. You must be their guide.

I was very privileged to have Joe and Clara Pilates and John Winters, Joe's right-hand man, as my first guides. None of them talked much. Joe liked to demonstrate and push and pull. I remember my first verbal correction which came after quite a few lessons, "Use your gut!" Clara liked to poke. "Dis," she would say as an arthritic finger jabbed into the muscle she wanted you to use. It sent an immediate message to the brain. No amount of talking could have conveyed as much information as that quick poke. John was, by nature, a quiet man. An organist by profession (no one earned a living teaching Pilates), he was actually quite shy. He would sit quietly, looking vaguely amused as he watched you perform your exercises, then offer one simple suggestion. "Try this." You tried and it practically killed you! He would giggle. But it changed the entire exercise, and you would have discovered something entirely new about your body.

I am often asked what it was like in Joe's original studio. After years of struggling to make people understand, I finally realized that it is one of those "you had to be there" things, like the last minute of the Super Bowl. To understand that studio, you have to understand the culture of the time. The world was a totally different place. There were no computers, no cell phones (but there were a lot of pay phones. Some of them even worked!). Records were kept by hand in journals and on index cards. People did not exercise unless they were athletes or dancers. If you saw someone running in Central Park, chances were there was a policeman running 25 feet behind him. People were passionate, responsible, and polite - not because of rules and regulations, they just were. Clients were addressed as Mr., Mrs. or Miss, not by first names.

And speaking of running, in 1967, the year that Joe died, a woman named Kathrine Switzer made headlines by being the first woman to run the Boston Marathon. Shocking. It was thought by many that if a woman exercised, she would grow hair on her chest and destroy her reproductive ability. Women were not officially allowed in the Marathon until 1974, and it was another 10 years before the women's marathon became part of the Olympics.

The exercise boom that most of you grew up with is really something quite new. I've learned how difficult it is for you to relate to the world of Joe's time. Napoleon once said, "If you want to understand a man, look at what the world was like when he was 20." In Joe's case, that was 1900ish. That is a real eye-opener.

People come to Pilates for many different reasons – sometimes sent by a doctor or physical therapist, sometimes to improve their golf or tennis game, sometimes just to improve their physical condition. As developed by Joe Pilates, it is a method of exercise. Very correct exercise. And very demanding exercise. Not only the whole body, but the mind must be engaged at all times.

But I am starting to see something missing. It should also be fun. Joe often talked about children and animals, the freedom, the joy in moving and discovering their bodies.

How many two- and three-year-olds have walked stark naked into a room full of company? Who is embarrassed? Not the child. It is always the parents with their rules and regulations and restrictive social mores. The child is simply doing what comes naturally and feels good.

Every child learns to walk in just about the same way. First they must learn to stand. How do they do that? What you think of as a coffee table is for the child a secret boost into the upright world. They learn that the table is stable and strong. They don't care why. As long as they can use it to pull that onerous body up off the floor, it is serving the purpose for which it was created. And after a number of attempts, voilà! Success! To celebrate, he slaps his hands on the table, promptly losing his balance, and falling back to the floor. So he tries again. Each attempt with a little more success. This is how the body learns. This is how muscles develop.

This is how Pilates works.

How do you teach a child to swing? With a lot of talk of anatomy and aerodynamics? Or do you just put him on the swing, push, and let nature take its course? Through the movement, the child quickly feels which muscles are working and what he must do to maintain his momentum. Job done! No explanation needed.

Again, this is how Pilates works.

I am sure you are all familiar with the "Six Principles of Pilates"and I am equally sure you all know they did not come from Joe. They come from a book published in 1980, thirteen years after Joe died. The intent was to distinguish Pilates from all the other forms of exercise that were becoming popular. And those principles are good. But for me, the most important principle is missing: MOVE! Change comes through movement, not talking. Just like the child on the swing, get moving and it is amazing how the body responds.

For me, Joe's true genius was how he built everything into his exercises. This is why you must have every exercise on every apparatus, large and small, in your own body. Then, and only then, will you be able to choose the right exercise for the body in front of you. You choose, get the body moving, and Joe will do the rest! This is the mark of a truly good Pilates teacher—knowing which exercise will address the issues of a particular body.

I am often asked, as I am sure you are, is Pilates good for this or that sport, will it help me with this or that activity, will I look better? The answer, of course is yes, yes, and yes. How is this possible? I like to think of the body as an instrument, let's say the piano.When you strike a key on the piano, through a series of mechanisms, a felt-covered hammer strikes a string or strings. The string or strings vibrate, creating a sound. As long as the piano is properly constructed, maintained, and tuned, this is how it works. The piano doesn't care if you are playing Bach or rock and roll; this is how it works. The only difference, in fact, between Bach and rock and roll is which keys are struck, the rhythm, and the dynamics. So too with the body. For a properly constructed and tuned body, the only difference between ballet and bowling is which combination of muscles is used, the rhythm and the dynamics. You are still playing the same instrument, just a different tune. I know I am simplifying this, but I think you get the idea.

People will be bad at the beginning. So was I. So were you. They have a right to be bad! You have to start where you are. If their bodies were perfect, they wouldn't need you. Dangerous should never be allowed, but bad is to be expected. Get used to it. It will get better if you allow it, which means allowing the client to find things in their own body. You wouldn't chastise a child for falling in his attempt to stand. You would encourage them to try again. Guide your clients through the right exercises for their particular bodies, and the results will come. But not in an hour or a week. We live in a culture of instant gratification, but Pilates is a process that takes time. Be patient, You are changing a lifetime of bad habits.

Know what you can do and be proud of your ability and accomplishments, but know your limits too. Completing the "Anatomy Coloring Book", no matter how beautifully you do it, is not a medical credential. I once heard a physical therapist, lamenting the minimal coverage provided by insurance companies, telling a group of Pilates teachers, "You must fill in the gap." I was horrified. We are not physical therapists! They have years of medical training, and we should not be encroaching on their territory.

There exists a lack of understanding and confusing information about what Pilates actually is. However, this misunderstanding is not just the provence of the general public. The medical profession is confused too. Many doctors think Pilates is another form of physical therapy. It is not! It is exercise. Very correct exercise, which is why so many people achieve health benefits from it. But it should never, repeat never, be identified as physical therapy. Many of the aches and pains and complaints that people have are simply the result of poor alignment and stress. That we can handle. Move them through the appropriate exercises, and they will get relief. But know your limits. You probably know more about exercise than your doctor does, but he knows a lot of other things that you do not. There is no shame in that. If you needed brain surgery, would you go to your wonderful gardner? We all have our specialities and areas of expertise. Stay within your boundaries.

Wherever you got your Pilates training, I am sure you were nit-picked to death. Everything was explained, discussed, the joy beaten out of every exercise. As it should be. You are training to be a teacher responsible for other people's bodies. You must be held to a higher standard than the once-a-week mat class client. But you shouldn't treat your clients the way you were treated. This is not the time to exact your revenge! For some of you, I am sure Pilates takes up all your waking (and perhaps sleeping) hours. For your clients, it takes up maybe one to three hours a week. They have lives outside of Pilates–jobs, family, all sorts of responsibilities, and interests. Have mercy on them. Make those few hours a week special and fun. Let them leave with a smile on their face and a spring in their walk. Then you will have done a good job!

Good luck, and good health!

Jay

About Jay:

Jay Grimes began his studies with Joe Pilates in the mid-sixties and after Joe's death continued with Joe's wife, Clara, for another 10 years until her death. Jay began teaching in the original 8th Ave studio in New York and has since taught all over the world. Jay danced professionally, ballet and Broadway for 18 years, and never had an injury. This he attributes entirely to Pilates. Jay is valued in the Pilates community for his experience, humility, and integrity in maintaining the work of Joe Pilates. Over the years, Jay's clients have ranged from stars of Broadway and Hollywood, music and opera to politicians, businessmen and housewives, and Olympic athletes.

The Core Connection

By Chris Robinson

You need a strong mind to guide your body; you need a strong body to follow your mind.

I will never forget my first Pilates lesson! It was back in the 1990s. Although I had heard of Pilates, I didn't really know much about it. Believing it was a combination of ballet and yoga, it didn't interest me much. But one of my kickboxing students, Michael Johnson, wanted to teach Traditional Pilates; he asked me for a tradeout - kickboxing lessons for Pilates lessons. I agreed. My first session with Michael was an Advanced Reformer workout. I remember thinking, *What on earth is he doing?* I mean, he was teaching what I thought were strange exercises. I was on this crazy apparatus. But it was really challenging and fun!

At first I thought, *This feels okay. And it's pretty interesting.* But as the workout progressed, I really began to see the value of the system. This was powerful stuff! An hour later, when I got off the Reformer, I felt instantly that I could punch and kick harder. I could move better. Pilates was like nothing I had ever done before. I was hooked.

It's not as if working out was new to me. I am a lifelong athlete. My fascination with sports started in my elementary school P.E. class. Since age five, I have competed in football, baseball, basketball and track and field. At age 14, I turned to martial arts, which I continue to practice today.

As a competitive athlete, winning is essential. To that end, I do everything possible to improve my performance. One of my biggest motivations for practicing Traditional Pilates technique is that this system of body conditioning makes me a better athlete. It teaches me how to move better; it prevents injury. When an athlete trains for or plays a sport, the body must successfully execute a variety of movements in spontaneous and rapidly changing circumstances. Any athlete can easily get injured because he is frequently moving outside the normal range of motion with rapidly changing weight load distributions. The traditional Pilates system teaches people how to correctly establish movement from The Center—or Powerhouse muscles—directing energy safely and effectively through the extremities with highly trained coordination.

Studying with Michael, I understood that traditional Pilates technique is a unique way to train muscles, practice alignment, and develop coordination from all the right places in the body. It is an intelligent and extremely challenging workout. Sadly though, I had only had four or five lessons with Michael when he relocated back to New York City. Before he left, he suggested, "If you really want to learn, go to New York and train with this lady, Romana Kryzanowska. She will really teach you The Work." I thought, *You know what, I see that there's a lot to this workout. Let me do this.* About six months later, Michael connected me to Moses Urbano to begin preparation for the Pilates education program. I worked with Moses for a few months. When he said I was ready, I made the move, relocating from San Diego to New York City to start teacher training with Romana. It was really a daring move to make; it took a lot of time and a lot of money. But I saw the value of understanding and teaching The Work. And this was just the beginning.

Coming from an athletic background and not really understanding Traditional Pilates technique at the beginning, I remember trying to "muscle through" everything. Training with Romana really taught me how to move from The Center and really develop core strength. That is something most people don't understand: establishing movement from the Powerhouse is a process that takes time, discipline, study, and expertise.

Fast-forward 15 years, and I continue to gain knowledge and skill about the traditional work, particularly as it applies to martial arts. There is always something deeper to learn in both disciplines. Although I've been doing martial arts for 30 years, I'm still learning techniques. With movements I already know, I learn how to improve them. After many years of studying and training, I'm really starting to understand where the power of my punch comes from; I'm connecting deeper from the Powerhouse when I kick in martial arts. It's the same with Pilates. Each time I train, I understand how to accomplish The Hundred a little more correctly. I don't think that will ever change. You never get to absolute perfection; but you always get closer and closer, deeper and deeper to that Powerhouse center and core of understanding.

Traditional Pilates technique teaches me how to stay "within the joint" no matter what extreme range of motion I put my body in. What I'm seeing with my teammates—a lot of other guys are really strong, but they're only strong in certain areas. They're not strong throughout the forward range of motion. When they force their bodies to those extreme ranges, usually they get injured. That used to happen to me all the time, but it's been quite a long while since I've been seriously injured in martial arts. Now, when I'm fighting, I'm actually thinking about Pilates and moving from my Powerhouse; it's definitely taken my martial arts to a higher level.

Here are the reasons why:

1) It keeps me from being injured so I can train more and improve martial arts technique;
2) I continue to deepen my knowledge of the body, where my strength comes from; and
3) I achieve the highest level of athletic ability possible. It will continue to take me years to move with a full Powerhouse connection and without extraneous tension; that's extremely important in Pilates, as well as in martial arts.

My obsession with understanding how to better execute different kinds of movement led me to pursue an academic degree in kinesiology. I wanted to understand biomechanics. Traditional Pilates breaks down exercises in useful ways. Now I can see common denominators of movement, the building blocks of everyday activity or skilled sports. There is important value in having this knowledge, especially since I have also worked as a personal trainer over the years. As a result, my clients accomplish physical activities more effectively and with better movement quality.

And it has enabled me to engage men's interest in Pilates. When they see me practice martial arts or participate in a sport, they immediately notice the strength I have developed, the ways I use it, and how I move. So I tell them that strength, flexibility, and fast reaction time come from traditional Pilates technique. This communication helps them understand the athletic benefits of The Work. As a result, there is potential for men to perceive this body conditioning system as effective, results-oriented, and legitimate. They think, *Okay, this guy can do it. Apparently this Pilates work enables him to move a certain way when he's fighting or playing a sport.* But it's a tough sell because a lot of men think that Pilates is for women; so it's hard for them to take their first lesson. I've told so many of my teammates, "Hey, guys, come and train with me. Let me give you a lesson. Let me show you what Traditional Pilates is." But they have their own ideas about The Work; again, they don't think it is challenging enough for men.

Men are most often drawn to the traditional system when they're injured. At this point, they realize they can't do their normal weight lifting routine or gym-based body conditioning workout. So they try Pilates and work really hard because that's their usual approach to exercise. They sweat and exert the same amount of effort as lifting heavy weights. And they feel like they're getting strong; but at the same time, when they're done, they feel good and they have symptom relief. The reason is that Traditional Pilates technique works all the muscles from the right place, while using the right amount of effort and strength. Once men realize they can get a vigorous workout without strain or pain, they can strengthen with vitality. Then they realize the value of Traditional Pilates.

When men lift weights, they often develop muscle tightness. They push their muscles to fatigue, often working too hard for optimal performance outside the gym. Some of their movement coordination and flexibility can be lost by gaining this strength. In addition, they often don't develop strength in the right muscle groups. This can limit their ability to achieve higher levels of physical skill in other activities.

Once men get past the misconception that traditional Pilates is for women, they can definitely develop strength and feel challenged in this great system of body conditioning, while increasing range of motion and coordination. They realize, *Wow, I can move faster, I can move freer.* Then men latch on; they appreciate and want to do The Work.

I'm teaching a couple of fighters now. They began with one lesson per week, quickly transitioning to twice a week. It wasn't long before they felt better, recognizing, *If I did this three times a week, man, I could really get a lot of benefit.* Now they train because they can't step away from it. They see the value. Just like myself. If I don't train in Pilates for a few weeks, my body doesn't feel right. Consistently doing The Work keeps everything in The Center; it gives relief to the body; it gives a freedom of movement that is unmatched in any other system. Once you understand that, you appreciate The Work. You have to dedicate yourself and it's a lifelong journey. There are so many ways to practice, train, and study that provide new information, body knowledge, and skill. You must keep your body and your mind conditioned by understanding The Work. The Traditional Pilates system is deep.

I'm fortunate to have an incredible teacher to guide me. I've been working with Jay Grimes for many years now, and every lesson I learn something completely new. I have also learned from my colleagues and friends, particularly Moses Urbano and Kathi Ross-Nash. And I observe other friends, like Brooke Siler, Dana Santi, and Peter Fiasca teaching workshops. Just as important in a different way, I learn from teaching my students. When I teach an exercise in a way that I never thought about before, I see something new or learn an important insight that contributes to the benefit of my students as well as my own knowledge. A year from now I'll look back and think, *Oh, my God, I've learned so much more since then.*

What an amazing journey Pilates has been and continues to be. When I first started, I wanted to really be connected, but didn't know how to work the Powerhouse and connect all the other muscles. So I just dug in deep and tensed my body to find that connection. What I have discovered is that too much tension decreases performance in any sport, martial art, or body conditioning. It's crucial to aim toward optimal distribution of energy. You want to be strong, but you want to move without tension. It's very challenging; it's the art of control. You need a strong mind to guide your body; you need a strong body to follow your mind. Sometimes you direct your body to accomplish a particular movement or series of movements, but it may not be strong enough or coordinated enough. You can develop enormous amounts of strength, but sometimes—if you have all that strength with no control—it is useless. Staying true to Traditional Pilates technique will keep you on the right path.

About Chris:

As a lifelong athlete, Chris Robinson is constantly in pursuit of peak performance. With great passion and energy, the Houston native brings that drive to the service of his clients, including Oprah Winfrey, for whom he acted as personal core coach. A certified Pilates instructor with more than 15 years of professional fitness experience, Chris learned his craft directly from Pilates legend Romana Kryzanowska as well as Jay Grimes.

Just Do It!

By Cynthia Lochard

> ***Navigating the balance between intense physical exertion and establishing technical correctness is extremely important.***

To accomplish Pilates at high levels with exact placement, alignment, balance, and line is an extremely difficult feat; and this is where many men lose interest in Pilates, unless they have studied gymnastics or martial arts. Most men like vigorous exercise. They like physical work. They like to move. For them, achieving ideal technical forms with the aim of perfection in Pilates is secondary, as it should be. Yet many Pilates teachers look for an ideal approach, a perfect technique, a textbook picture of how the body should look, unwittingly creating a source of discontent for most male students. Instead, we should teach men a strong foundation of athletic movement, achieving a balance between body-brain strength and development of knowledge.

It's important to make a distinction between pushing "gung ho" to get a vigorous, athletic workout and developing a strong physical foundation, as well as an understanding of your body. Too often, teachers focus on perfect Pilates technique—the perfect Footwork, the perfect Hundred. The intention of creating correct exercise shapes with alignment, placement, and energy certainly has great merit. Yet instructors often focus on these aspects of Traditional Pilates at the expense of teaching strong athletic movement. This limitation can hold students back from achieving the full benefits of Joe Pilates' system, unwittingly depriving them of the remarkable results that come from moving vigorously and athletically. Many teachers are waiting for students to achieve exacting technical forms before they can experience exhilarating movement and tackle the serious challenge of developing optimal mental and physical conditioning. Too many students are limited by these well-intentioned, knowledgeable teachers. They would be better served by striving for a balance between vigorous, coordinated, flexible strength, and "correct" form.

There are a lot of different dynamics in Traditional Pilates; nowadays, though, so much Pilates education and training is based on safety, safety, safety first, which prevents people from taking reasonable risks or maintaining a work ethic of vigorous conditioning. This is reflected in how men are taught. Women teachers often don't fully understand this balance between teaching "corrective exercise" and vigorous movement. Unfortunately, they teach men in a sort of remedial way, instead of just letting them figure it out as they go along.

There is definitely a different dynamic between the emotional state of the man compared to a woman, particularly when it comes to the body. Most men are more interested in just feeling something and then understanding it afterwards, but many women teachers try to achieve the goals of alignment and placement before they encourage athletic movement. And few women can accomplish the highest levels of Classical Pilates training. Kathi Ross-Nash performs The Work much like a very advanced male, yet she is clearly feminine. Not many women have that rare kind of physical strength or clear mental intention. Both areas are essential; however, there's a big difference between the two. Romana navigated the balance by encouraging people to move while correcting them along the way. She inspired us to move to the limits of our capabilities; if we were approaching our limit, then we knew it. As a teacher, you will never know how far is too far if you don't allow someone to try.

When I first began learning Traditional Pilates, the training was hard. Two of my early teachers were sweet guys, but there was no nonsense. They just focused and made me do The Work. Their approach was "full on," which is, ironically, why I didn't have full appreciation of Pilates at the time; it was very hard work right from the beginning. As I gained more experience, I began to understand more of Joe Pilates' system. He knew that most men are not capable of, nor are they interested in, making perfect lines and perfect shapes. Men want to move; men want to work. Yet they need to learn "corrective exercise," as Joe Pilates described, to increase safety by improving stability, coordination, flexibility, stamina, and peak physical performance. That's what many women Pilates teachers don't understand.

My training with Romana and Sari was equally as demanding. The certification program was fairly new, so there weren't many apprentices enrolled. Often, the only other apprentice in the studio was Peter

Roël from the Martha Graham Dance Company. When we had free time, we worked out together, and Romana often played with us. As I became stronger, she made me do things that Peter was capable of doing; of course, I didn't think twice about it. I just took the challenge. Then she would giggle and say, "But you may only teach that exercise to men." I often thought, *Oh, damn, I'm never going to do that again.* It was an interesting approach because I learned how to be safe without being pedantic or too cautious.

This early training shaped my attitude toward The Work and its approach, which differs markedly from the way it is taught today. When I first started teaching, I had a certain attitude about The Work and its approach, different from what we're teaching today. I worked in an area called Leichhardt, a predominantly Italian area in Sydney. Because I was a dancer, I taught a lot of dancers. But my work as a teacher also developed through referrals from a physical therapist. The majority of clients were men, so I was fortunate to have this practical experience. First of all, we didn't have as much information in the program as we tend to give out these days. Second, a lot of the men were sports enthusiasts and professionals. It was important to approach the traditional Pilates work in a way that kept them interested because it was very beneficial for them. So I approached The Work from a more emotional place. For example, I referred to Ballet Stretches as Footy Stretches because I was watching the Footy Game. I could see the guys on the sidelines doing the same stretches on the ladder rungs. But they would never make that connection. And, of course, I could then sneak in a few extra details like placement, alignment, lift, mental focus, and a little analysis to grow their interest. And I still have those clients today. That was 22 years ago.

Although it's harder work for a woman to teach men, it's certainly very interesting. There is a sense in which I don't have to be as careful with them. As teachers-in-training, we were not encouraged to do so much spotting. We were taught The Work and we observed how Romana and Sari worked with different body types; we just developed a certain level of intuition. Romana would say, "Use common sense." As apprentices, we developed an understanding of The Work. Then we were able to rely upon this common sense and adapt our teaching as necessary or desirable to the individual. In the words of Romana, when teaching a client, "The Method is right in front of you."

In more recent years, there are clearly more concerns about technique, care, and safety—to the point of almost fearing the body. This is the opposite of what Joe Pilates intended; he wanted people to become confident as a result of increasing strength, coordination, flexibility, and concentration. The body is indeed resilient; it's the mind that can develop restraints and fear and various complications. Students are being held back from achieving their full potential and highest level of capability. Although some clients may eventually reach their goals, it's taking a lot longer compared to when Romana was teaching. When you're working with men, this can be a problem because they can't feel the vigorous traditional work.

The focus of my work with clients is embodied in one question, "What is this body capable of achieving?" I remain within the framework of implications that arise from this question. I will push a man physically, in literal ways—strongly physically stretching, pulling, pressing—as well as in figurative ways. Perhaps I would not approach a five-foot female who weighs 90 pounds in the same way; but she has other challenges, so I would work with a different approach. I am careful with all students. Since I'm very intuitive, I can sense when movement might be going too far rather than not going far enough. It's important that people exert themselves as much as they possibly can. Students have to develop strength and stamina to improve The Work and technique. After teachers guide students to improve their work and technique, then we should take them beyond. They will not have the stamina to sustain high levels of technique with complete correctness anyway. Navigating the balance between intense physical exertion and establishing technical correctness is extremely important. Striking the best balance—even a good balance—is often missing. That affects the difference between teaching women and men because they feel The Work differently. Basically, men are stronger, but they have more muscle tightness in their bodies. Although I don't know how a man feels Traditional Pilates, if I were to be too specific about holding him back or not letting him move because his technique is not sufficiently correct, he would lose interest. Men just need to move. There are, of course, common areas of the body wherein both men and women benefit from Traditional Pilates technique.

Everybody can gain mental and physical conditioning from Classical Pilates. Certainly, women's bodies can be a bit more fragile, a little more delicate. They may have had three children, for instance, in which case, their pelvic bones are different from a man's. As a result of those differences, the way in which you address them should be different too, even if just slightly. There is an emotional aspect as well. Some men are a little uncomfortable taking instruction from a female who's providing information about their abilities and limitations. This gender difference can be a sensitive issue. All in all, though, it's psychologically important for students to understand how special this work is, how the vigor and complexity of Joe Pilates' integrated system is so personally beneficial. And it's a lot of fun to work with men! Why? Because you just go for it! You don't have to be so mindful about, oh, this, that, and the other thing. In this respect, it takes a little bit less effort; in another sense, it's a bit harder because they're bigger, heavier. You've got to put in a lot of energy when you're working with men. As a teacher, when you have eight male students in a given day, it can be exhausting, particularly if they need the assisted Bicycle on the Cadillac.

Currently, I am teaching a man whose name is Michael; he is a professor in his 60s, and his body is extremely tight. Without a doubt, I work him just as hard as I would any man who is very fit. But there are specific exercises that I don't give him because they would intensify his body's inflexibility. With other exercises, I reduce range of motion; but again, I teach Michael as vigorously as anyone. I push him to the limits of his capability, which is the point I have been making. I don't hold back with anyone, male or female. I am fortunate to understand when I can teach students beyond their own perceived abilities; it takes dedication and many years to know when it's beneficial to push someone "to the wall." But I go "to the wall," and that's far enough. I'm careful not to go beyond; it would be too much. Students tend to derive a great deal of benefit from this positive exertion, increased skill and accomplishment; it's a place they're not willing or capable of taking themselves. I teach students to perform at 150% or more of their perceived capability. Otherwise, it's a waste of time; they can go somewhere else for that.

Allowing people to move, teaching them to take risks, giving them space, supporting their courage, and not handling them too much are all very important. Of course, as a teacher, it's also important to be close enough in case the student needs your assistance, even if that is emotional. Just letting them do The Work is best. It's frustrating to see how careful and restrictive The Work has become. I don't comply with this trend, and I certainly don't enjoy seeing it happen. It's boring! And it does not offer people the best form of conditioning. In striking contrast, it was athletic and gymnastic intensity that defined Joe Pilates' system of conditioning, as well as the formidable technique of his entire system; it's what set Romana apart from other teachers and other modalities.

I hold true to Romana's values of teaching movement; it certainly makes the process easier, more fun and more tangible for students. When someone is moving, it's a lot easier to see where he is strong and where he is weak. For example, you might be able to hold your foot in alignment if you're barely moving. Through any range of motion, though, if you change placement or alignment, ask these questions: Can you still articulate the foot in a biomechanically correct way? Can you stabilize in the right places and stay aligned in the right places while generating optimum energy with full awareness from head to toe? In essence, that's what makes The Work fun and challenging.

The U.S. is similar to Australia: predominantly women teach or practice The Work. Nontraditional Pilates is relatively remedial, promoted as a kind of noninvasive, meditative activity. So men never developed an interest in Pilates unless they happened to know someone who teaches the real work. On the other hand, in Latin American countries and throughout Europe, more men train in Pilates. Over the years, men have certainly been training at my studio; the success is primarily due to word of mouth. We teach corporate classes, comprised largely of men, and that draws attention to the studio. We also teach classes at the opera house; these attract a lot of stagehands who have injuries or just don't feel in optimal physical condition because they work late at night and then they carry heavy equipment the entire next day. So they attend classes and slowly they get involved. I've also had a lot of male students from different walks of life who promote Traditional Pilates to their friends.

And so, over the years, we've just developed a good balance in clientele as a natural result of teaching the Traditional Pilates system and having an excellent reputation. I don't do any sort of direct promotion. However, we always explain that the system of body conditioning was developed by a strong athletic man. I talk a lot about the history of Joe Pilates - that he developed his work from being a tough gymnast, boxer, martial artist, and circus performer. The more people I teach over the years, the more genius I see in his work; and I always share those revelations, those insights with my clients and with my teachers. People really enjoy it. I appreciate Joe's legacy, what he "left behind for the world," as he puts it. It is heartening to see the wider community "humbling up" and working together to keep the traditional system in its entirety. Each teacher possesses little parts of the whole; let's acknowledge that and preserve the whole by seeing all of its parts.

About Cynthia:

Born in New York City, Cynthia Lochard began learning The Pilates Method in 1976 as a young dancer. Later, she received a contract to dance with the New York City Ballet and worked for some of the world's greatest choreographers, like George Balanchine and Jerome Robbins and others. During this time, she continued to practice Pilates at the then Joseph Pilates studio in New York City with Romana Kryzanowska. Cynthia brought the first Authentic Teacher-Training program to Sydney in 1998. During this time she continued to travel back to NYC to participate in further developing what is now known as Romana's Teacher Training Program, now more commonly referred to as the "Classical" training. In 2009, Romana appointed Cynthia one of only three Master Teacher Trainers worldwide. Cynthia has trained most of the true classical Pilates instructors operating throughout Australia, Asia, New Zealand, United States, and Russia.

The Body Says What Words Cannot

By Fredrik Prag

Traditional Pilates technique gives men time to reflect, learn, and transform.

Teaching Traditional Pilates to men is all about encouraging them to move with strength and coordination; it is not about verbal correction. For men, learning the technique is about moving and being. When a man doesn't know anything about Classical Pilates, I introduce The Work by guiding his movement with very little or no verbal instruction. Although it's a teacher's responsibility to verbally correct movement, there is a point of diminishing returns; it's better to listen to the student's body through visual observation. As he moves, I get the information of what he is communicating. If I exert too much presence, I block his natural growth and who he is, expressed through movement.

There is a necessary gap—between silent guidance and verbal correction—for the purpose of providing the most positive educational experience. When I teach men, I step away and create some distance. There is a sense in which I'm not really there. This affords the male student educational and transformational space. Of course, I guide him to properly accomplish movement forms, to recognize what it feels like when he moves correctly. These feelings then guide the body to make shapes and develop technique. At first, he may be uncoordinated and misaligned, but it's okay. He needs to move; he needs to move for about 50 minutes. If The Work in his body has only made marginal progress a year later, that's okay, too!

As teachers, we can't explain how to move because it's too complicated. Movement and language are qualitatively different realms. When I see a man practice Pilates movements, I sometimes think to myself, *Oh, he's doing this wrong. He's doing that wrong. He doesn't understand anything.* But I just shut up; I do not speak. It may take months or even years before he wakes up, gradually achieving more physical and mental conditioning in the Traditional Pilates system. But his body and his mind will "become" Pilates.

Teaching Pilates is a deep experience for students and teachers. Men walk into the studio with certain expectations. They expect to look physically strong, which is primarily defined by gaining large muscle mass, losing fat, and performing to fatigue. Due to worldwide commercial media stereotypes and images of ideal masculinity, as well as corporate interest in selling various so-called health foods for increased physical performance, men feel pressured, often unconsciously, to achieve these ideals.

When a man starts to work out, he expects to fatigue himself by achieving peak performance. Although I no longer train at the physical level of professional sports, I understand men generally have this expectation for themselves. Their quest for physical performance comes with significant limitations; they are not interested in mental conditioning, let alone developing a spiritual connection. By spiritual, I mean a sense of creativity, a sense of being open to transformation without changing Joe Pilates' technique. Since most men are not interested in connecting to mental/spiritual aspects of movement, teachers can help them connect by emphasizing what they already know: (1) if a man expects to get tired, make him tired; (2) if he expects strenuous peak performance, demand strenuous peak performance; (3) if he expects endurance, require protracted stamina during every workout. If instructors do not connect to men's expectations and self-perceptions, men will never continue in the Pilates system.

Although we don't think in terms of targeting or isolating muscles in Traditional Pilates technique, it's useful to help clients focus their conscious work effort in ways that feel familiar and good, yet do not make them feel or look uncoordinated. A man's resilience and confidence often camouflage an unexpectedly sensitive side. In my opinion, this is because he has not achieved more informed mental or spiritual conditioning. As a teacher, my job is to guide him on his journey, so we start working with the physical. But one doesn't get there overnight. I taught one man for over two years before he reached improved mental understanding. Only then could he begin developing his spirit within aspects of physical and mental conditioning.

Originally the man didn't know why he wanted to study traditional Pilates. Then one day he remarked, "Wow, Fredrik, this lesson hour, it's the highlight of the week." As his teacher, I knew the man was starting to change because the Pilates system was gradually becoming more conscious. In the beginning, the student's body and spirit were groping in the dark; they were seeking evolution. When the man's brain began to achieve a higher threshold of reflection and better understand the process, that's when he became more responsive and engaged. And that's when I start to increase my verbal instruction with men. Of course none of this would be possible without Joe Pilates' brilliant integrated system of movement.

Recently I had the opportunity to teach two brothers who competed at European-level mixed martial arts. They are between ages 20 and 25 and quite famous in their niche. Their bodies are in peak athletic form. All athletes have the same urge to become aligned, to improve, to feel better, to perform better. As a teacher, you might think there's not much to improve upon. Yet the Traditional Pilates Method helped these men become less physical, so to speak, by optimizing energy output as well as improving their mental/spiritual understanding of movement. If I had verbally corrected these men too much in the beginning, they would never have returned for Pilates training. They would never have changed for the better. Teaching the traditional system of Pilates is very powerful. When teachers talk less, it allows athletes to grow and achieve peak performance. It's due to me shutting up, really. So, too, it is important to take care of myself as a teacher communicating knowledge and exerting energy.

In the beginning, it was a challenge teaching top-level martial arts men. I pushed them with all the physically difficult advanced Pilates exercises. They did all the standing arm exercises with Cadillac leg springs, the full Wunda Chair, advanced Mat, standing exercises on the Reformer as well as acrobatic exercises on the Cadillac. Yet I never neglected Joe Pilates' ideas about movement, health, mental conditioning, corrective exercises, and athletic achievement. This combination of teaching physically difficult advanced exercises with Joe Pilates' philosophy intrigued these two athletes. They became inspired as a result of seeing the gap between brute strength and mental/spiritual presence within the body. This was my opportunity to explore this connection and increase athletic prowess. I taught these two brothers for approximately eight months. As time progressed, they began to see more value in exercises perceived as more fundamental: Footwork, The Hundred, Short Box Series, Leg Circles, Rolling Like a Ball, Stomach Massage Series, Push Through, Roll Back, Series of Five, and so forth. These men began to practice Pilates technique using Pilates movement, instead of relying upon force from lifting weights and explosive speed in mixed martial arts. They were connecting the physical with the mental/spiritual.

As a former athlete myself, I know it's essential to work with full power yet remain very still in your mind. When you teach exercises to any athlete, that individual should feel and exhibit inner stillness without tension, trying, wanting, or willing. He simply embodies movement. This is when he becomes more aligned physically, mentally and spiritually; there is concordance between embodying our full humanity and becoming more fully human.

As a kid, I loved to move. And running was my passion. Most of all, I enjoyed running fast. But I always wondered, *Could I run even faster?* I had to find out. There was an athlete named Mike Powell who was competing at the same time as Carl Lewis. I was so impressed with Powell. To paraphrase, he once said, "You know, I have a masseur, I have a physical therapist, I have my personal coach, I have a manager, and I have a mental coach." He worked with all these professionals to achieve success. At first I thought, *I don't have those people; so how can I succeed? I'll just make my own way.* But I soon realized the wisdom of his words. I began to look for a masseur, a running coach, and an advisor, who all helped to improve my athletic performance. After many years of training and competing in track and field events, I reached my goal of running 100 meters in 10.5 seconds. During this time period, I had creative forces that pushed me into learning how to run faster. I studied biomechanics, plyometrics, speed, weight lifting, nutrition, "explosive" sports training, corrective exercise, balance—everything to learn more and perform better. Although I competed at high levels, I never really enjoyed it, and I'm not sure why. Yet I developed an interest in body conditioning and mental conditioning techniques.

When I encountered the Pilates system, it triggered something in my subconscious. There was no competition. I thought, *Finally, I can move without competing.* There was no stage where I had to perform with utmost speed. There was only me, the Mat, my body, and my ability. It was impossible to win or to lose or show off. Although the 100 meter race is about showing off, this was never my intention in running a race. So, Traditional Pilates corresponded to values I believed in; it's an original method of movement without external circumstances pushing you in a specific direction. Traditional Pilates makes you feel good; it helps you sustain healthy, functional movement and prepares you for any physical activity. These qualities are very good for men.

On the surface, however, we are confronted with a paradox: society trains men to think and act competitively, but the Pilates system is not competitive. The resolution of this paradox, of course, is that a man can compete within himself to achieve improved technique and mental conditioning; he is not competing against other men in the traditional Pilates system. Yet the competitive mentality is strongly instilled; that's one reason why so few men develop an interest in Pilates. For men, competition is everywhere and there is little choice. In contrast, women seem to study Pilates to explore their creativity as well as improve functional fitness. There are exceptions, in my observations, but Pilates constitutes creative expression for women and competitive expression for men. Although I do my best to transform the competitive mindset of men, it's the system of Traditional Pilates technique that naturally achieves this goal, in addition to developing a very strong, healthy, coordinated, and athletic physique. The additional reward for men is that Pilates is excellent for competition outside the studio. If you like to compete in martial arts, boxing, skiing, running, swimming, tennis, or any other physical activity, go to competitions—and win!

I have some high achieving professional men who come to the studio. Their whole day is occupied with achieving monetary and material success. They're pushed into these types of competitions due to circumstances and societal values. These men may work in finance or other high-risk competitive ways of making a living. As they arrive in the studio, they are in a competitive mode mentally, physically and spiritually. As teachers, we can help these men channel their competitive urges. Give them the Pull Up exercise on the Wunda Chair (with one spring). Although this lower spring setting will result in frustration and bad form, it will generate more respect and intrigue for the

Pilates system. After the client experiences the serious challenge, then you, as an instructor, can assist him by holding the hips and lifting him up while he directs his energy into the Wunda Chair apparatus. It's beneficial for men to understand the amount of Powerhouse strength required to properly execute Pilates exercises. This will not hurt men in Pilates. Yet executing strenuous movements in the gym can potentially cause injuries when using dumbbells or practicing deep squats with barbells. Within the Pilates system, men can push their frustration and ambition into all exercises. As time progresses, their frustration becomes more of a natural energy they can harness and use wisely.

With our previous Wunda Chair exercise in mind, let us consider springs more specifically. Using springs in any range of motion allows us to consider questions about initiating movement, distributing energy, correcting alignment, developing coordination, establishing dynamic balance, gaining stamina, articulating shape, and many other elements of movement. Because of the complexities involved in establishing movement quality and increasing body responsiveness, springs give men and women time to reflect upon their Pilates technique. Yet for men, this is very important because when they compete, there is little or no time for this reflection in the competitive mindset. Men are habitually focused on competition because their perceived or actual survival could be at stake. Competition means that somebody's interested in pushing you down. So you need to be ready. Traditional Pilates technique gives men time to reflect, learn, and transform. This is an opportunity for them to develop openness, skill, preparedness, quality of movement, and higher quality of life. Reflection starts to enlighten the brain. Questions can be asked. Using springs helps men work with Pilates apparatus to meet and explore dynamics of resistance and translate it within themselves instead.

Coming from a world of competition, men develop more creativity and their own space to explore, replenish, and thrive. But it's important to train in the entire method with all apparatus and Mat. That's why Joe Pilates made his system of conditioning complete. He understood the rigidness of the manly brain and societal expectations, creating all the apparatus to really bend the mind and attitude of the man. Otherwise, he'll get bored; and you can trick him because he's not so smart in the beginning!

And The Method bends the mind and the attitude in other ways. As a man gains mastery in the technique, there may come a time when it is beneficial for the teacher to break down an exercise, refining the movement. This should be done decisively, with authority. However, the client may construe it as an attack on his ego, a reflection on his masculinity. It may even reduce him to tears. Despite the embarrassment or sense of vulnerability he may experience, this approach can help him gain insight into the breadth and depth of his personality, touching on areas within his mental and spiritual realms that he has never before encountered. Breaking down exercises often means breaking down the individual. Yet, he's capable of surmounting this challenge; he will make it. The feeling of temporary inadequacy soon gives way to true humility and a desire for growth and transformation.

This is all part of the Pilates journey. Joe explains it best: "By reawakening thousands and thousands of otherwise ordinarily dormant muscle cells, Contrology correspondingly reawakens thousands and thousands of dormant brain cells, thus activating new areas and stimulating further the functioning of the mind."

About Fredrik:

Fredrik Prag trained and studied as an apprentice for three years in Pilates Scandinavia's studio on Atlasgatan in Stockholm. Further studies followed in True Classical Pilates by Master Teacher Jay Grimes, Peter Fiasca, Moses Urbano, Cary Regan, Michael Rooks and others. For 13 years, Fredrik actively focused on professional athletics within highly established clubs such as Tureberg and Hellas; earning a place as one of the top 10 at 100m in Sweden. He is also a trained kinesiologist at the The Swedish Kinesiology School and has completed further studies at the Ackemann Institute.

Chapter II

Reflections on Teaching: A Male and Female Perspective

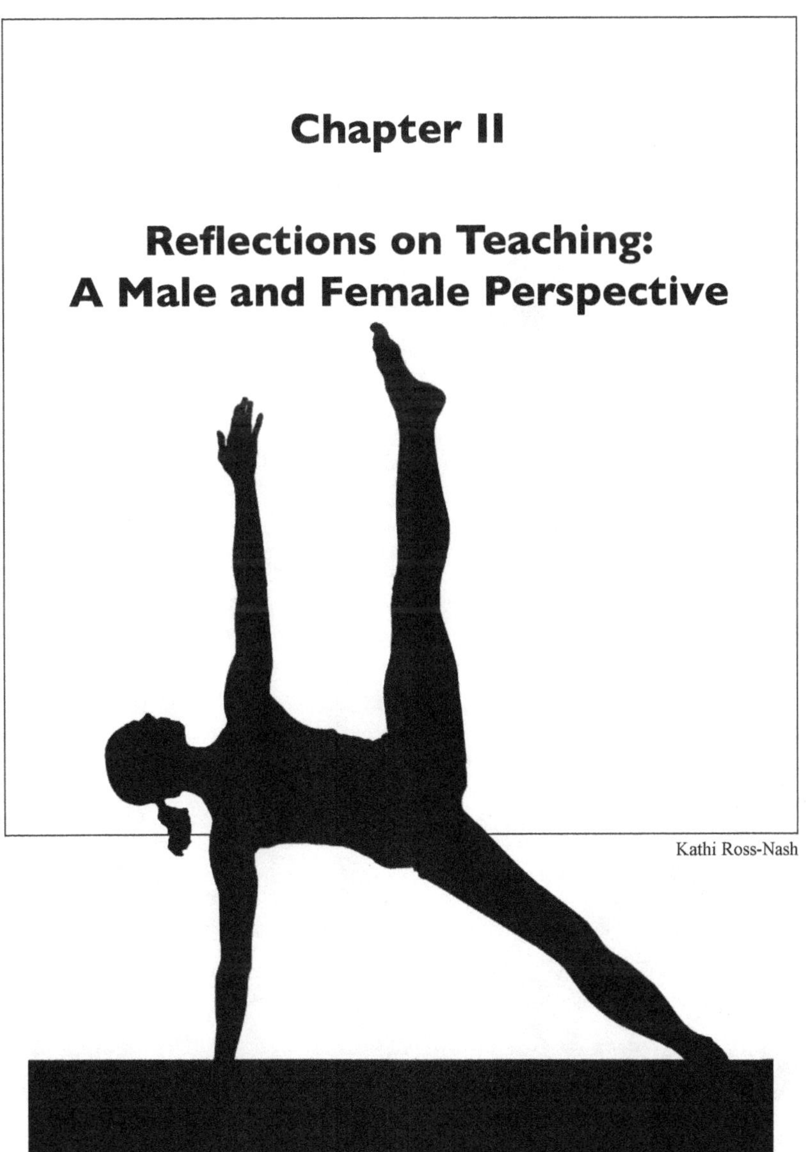

Kathi Ross-Nash

Growing up with Pilates

By Kathi Ross-Nash & Zak Ross-Nash

It was a blessing to know how to condition my body for sports.

KATHI: Being my first child, Zak began Pilates from the get-go. When he was a baby, we sometimes practiced little Teaser exercises together; we were like the original Mommy and Me duo. I actually did the Roll Up and Teaser with Zak on my leg and made it a game. When he was young, I observed his natural movement while he played outside in the yard, noticing what his body could naturally accomplish in terms of developing balance, agility, coordination, stability, strength and alignment. As his natural abilities developed, that movement guided my teaching. In Pilates, there is no set timetable that applies to every child; you can never say, "Okay, you're 12 years of age, practice this Pilates exercise on this apparatus." Every child develops differently according to his unique abilities and readiness to try new physical actions. I don't think Zak used the Electric Chair until he was in high school.

When Zak began karate, his first formal training, I became involved teaching Pilates at the karate studio. I incorporated Pilates Mat exercises into the warm-up of the karate class. In that way, Zak experienced a very organic exposure to Pilates. I never formally introduced The Work, saying, "This is the Pilates Method." I just presented it as exercise. When Zak started training in Pilates more consistently during the fifth grade, he worked out with apparatus; it was a very natural progression. There's a sense in which he grew up surrounded by the Traditional Pilates system. But I never said, "Oh, you're going to come do Pilates." Many exercises had already been part of his karate warm-up without calling them Pilates. Then when the time was right, I began teaching him apparatus work in my Pilates studio. I also drove Zak and my daughter, Zoe, to Drago's Gym in New York City when I trained with Romana. She loved both Zak and Zoe. Romana played with them! They were filmed with her for DVDs, and Zak participated in an extraordinary Pilates demonstration with Romana at Drago's.

So, he experienced Pilates from the beginning before he understood it was the greatest system of body conditioning ever!

ZAK: As far back as I can remember, I've been around Pilates. The technique wasn't ever forced; it was something that I grew up with, something familiar. I enjoyed doing it, in part, because I was around my mom and her friends. But I always benefited physically from The Work. Since I was a kid, I've always been physically active. I like to work out and play sports. My first vivid memory of practicing Pilates was at the karate studio where I trained, although at the time I didn't actually realize I was doing Pilates. My mom had come along for the day. We began our warm-up exercises, and she started teaching class. I thought, *All right, I'm just going to get down on the mat and do it; I'll try it out.* I really enjoyed the physical work, and I've been doing Pilates ever since.

I've played sports throughout my life. When I was younger, I wrestled, played football and baseball. I just finished my senior year of college football which has been intense. But many of my teammates regularly suffered pulled muscles, strains and other injuries, largely because they failed to consistently condition their bodies. Fortunately, I didn't experience these kinds of injuries; my muscles were limber and long, even though I'm somewhat of a stocky guy. The reason? I have been practicing Pilates for as long as I can remember. Sure, I've had bumps and bruises: I've broken my hand, sprained an ankle, and torn the labrum in my shoulder. During one game, I experienced hamstring pain after getting hit hard, falling in a certain way after a tackle.

KATHI: It's important to understand that Zak's injuries weren't from overly repetitive movement or incorrect action; the particular physical traumas he endured resulted from unavoidable circumstances like getting hit hard in a football game or being in a car accident. His torn labrum happened during a game on a particularly rainy evening. Another player tackled Zak hard; the way that he landed on his shoulder caused the injury. It was unavoidable. Injuries like that are impossible to prevent. Yet, it's important to consider what didn't happen: Zak was hit in the head, but he didn't injure his neck. As a running back, every time he had the ball, he was hit by multiple players. The fact that he has played football for 13 years and still has healthy knees, ankles, hips and a strong flexible back is due to Zak's diligence and the intelligence of Joe Pilates' integrated system of conditioning.

ZAK: When my labrum was partially torn playing football in high school, doctors specifically mentioned that my shoulder was very stable and flexible; that was why it didn't completely rip. There was a 90-degree tear in one area and a 180-degree tear in another area. The orthopedist noted that if I hadn't been in excellent physical condition, the labrum would have completely torn off. That would have set me back a long time in terms of preparing for college sports. It was a blessing to know how to condition my body for sports.

KATHI: When Zak was younger, he didn't have the alignment awareness to understand what his body needed. He had flat feet; very high, tight hips; significant lordosis; a tight upper back; and a soldier's neck. So I developed a training program for his needs. He practiced Mat and Reformer, then Arm Springs, pushups and jumping rope. At the time, he was running a lot, so he needed foundational Pilates work for flexibility. I started teaching Zak many exercises on the Cadillac, Electric Chair and Wunda Chair. When he was better able to understand the concept of alignment and the Pilates Method in general, he began achieving what Joe Pilates called mental conditioning or concentration; this is requisite in order to improve physical technique, coordination and responsiveness. Zak's mental desire and capacity were central to increasing physical skill. As an instructor, it's essential to effectively communicate with each student or client. If you teach young boys and you say, "Hold your hip in this position; don't rotate your arm; stabilize your back; externally rotate your thighs," the boys won't understand and may never want to learn Pilates. Look at their physical actions and encourage exercises that are interesting as well as fun. Let them naturally exert their muscles, learn, test their limits, and enjoy The Work for short periods of time to sustain interest and concentration; then go play outside the studio!

ZAK: Here are the coolest ideas I eventually came to understand: (1) there are fundamental Powerhouse muscle connections being used in all Pilates exercises; and (2) you can practice a single exercise on every apparatus in the studio. Once someone understands these points, Pilates becomes applicable and transferable to sports outside the studio. Inside the studio, I could translate any exercise to different apparatus, which meant that if I weren't activating abdominals on the Reformer, then I was ineffectively practicing the same way on the Barrels, the Wunda Chair or Cadillac. Having this understanding of the Pilates system translated into mental and physical adaptability and increased strength.

KATHI: Zak was the original Red Thread. Sometimes I show Zak's football photos to my students for educational purposes and ask them to look at his alignment and placement, identifying which Pilates exercises are informing his position. For example, in the Pilates studio, it was beneficial for Zak to frequently practice the Crossover Pumping exercise. Think about why: it's because he is frequently "cutting" in football. In the cutting action, players want to decelerate as quickly as possible to provide more time before pivoting and propelling in another direction. The pelvis is off balance, yet players are moving from the off-angle position of the hip. He also practiced Going Up Front on the Electric Chair and Wunda Chair for driving through on the football field and Going Up Side for quickly shifting side to side on the field. So, when my students look at Zak's photos, I ask them to consider this particular football player's function. Is he a linebacker? If so, he has to push on the field; he has to "move off." In Pilates, a linebacker could improve strength and coordination by practicing the Fencing exercise or Pilates pushups with one hand on the Wunda Chair pedal. The purpose is to understand the physical function by analyzing biomechanical actions that athletes must perform. Then we can teach Pilates exercises to strengthen those actions. When you're training an athlete, it's crucial to assess the needs for that particular athlete, not just balance and strengthen the body in general. Otherwise, a teacher will be committing the same error as making a ballerina "tight" because she already has flexibility. That's ridiculous; ballerinas must keep their flexibility and develop more strength within that flexibility.

As an instructor, you have to teach the body in front of you. You can't baby young athletes. Of course, if they have injuries, that's an entirely different story. But when you have a healthy body, just teach the exercises Joe Pilates provided, and use his Method to educate the person. Give them a strong full workout using studio apparatus. Don't teach a list of exercises; teach the body. If you're teaching a strong body, work it diligently, strengthen what is weak and challenge what is strong. Teachers often forget that very important point. We tend to say, "Oh, well they need this and they need that." No, look at that body. Can it do this? Yes. Is it pretty? Maybe not. Who cares? I can't imagine that Joe Pilates, a redneck German, did pretty work. Remember first and foremost that this is exercise. This is body conditioning; move your students, move your clients. Give them a workout because that's what they need.

One potential limitation of football coaching personnel is that, in the past, they often didn't sufficiently analyze the biomechanics of each football player's position on the field. They certainly focused on the importance of building muscle mass, which is useful, yet only part of the picture. If you evaluate football training over the years, the biomechanics of each player's position hasn't significantly improved, although there are some exceptions. At Stanford University, there is a functional sports trainer. And they're changing the program, individually analyzing each exercise for its usefulness in relation to the player's position on the field.

ZAK: What is the most important benefit of Pilates for me? It's the fact that I am strong and flexible. The combination of strength and flexibility enables me to fulfill my potential on the football field. It is the best way to identify and engage muscles I previously didn't know how to use. Now I know when I'm taking the ball over the goal line, not only am I driving with my legs, but I'm working abdominals to support driving forward with my back and arms. I initiate all muscle effort from The Center. Then I distribute it through the body to move forward on the football field. Pilates has given me the right tools to use my whole body while playing sports instead of activating separate, individual muscle groups. I'm not isolating limbs. All muscles work together.

KATHI: Zak's body conditioning was systemic, not reductionist; he trained his body as a whole, not in separate parts. When you look at any sports photos, you see many men and women working their upper bodies independent of their lower bodies. Through the lens of Traditional Pilates, it is clear there's no connection from the Powerhouse muscles (abdominals, inner thighs, lower back, inner thighs, gluteals) through the arms, legs, and head. It's precisely that connection, throughout the body in its entirety, that allows you to move with optimal coordination, dynamic balance, strength and control.

ZAK: The coaches and players on my team have begun to shift their focus from building as much bulk as possible to developing a combination of strength, flexibility, and speed. To that end, my teammates have experimented with different kinds of body conditioning techniques. Some tried yoga; others, like me, study Pilates. As a result, drastic improvements have been made. We've gone from a sub-500 record to 8-1, among the top 25 football teams in the country. This is awesome. I've shown my friends the science and art of Traditional Pilates. They realize that it's actually difficult to practice The Work the right way, but my friends keep coming back. Why? Because they get a great workout, and it keeps them playing football.

KATHI: My work with Zak's college football team has been minimal; it's just an introduction. I simply exposed the football players to a method of training that helps them prevent injuries, develop strength and flexibility, so they enjoy The Work. For young men who are interested in learning more, Zak takes his friends to Dana Santi's studio, The Pilates Core, or he practices Mat with them. I was more involved with Zak's high school football team, often going to the field to practice workouts with them, and I often invited the boys to my Pilates studio American Body Tech. Some of Zak's high school friends went on to play at Yale, Nuremberg, Franklin & Marshall. They all went on to have successful four-year college football careers, which is fantastic. For me, it was most important these young men continued to be successful.

I'm eternally grateful that Zak has grown up with an open mind; he has trusted me. I did not allow him to lift weights during his high school football career. As a mom, I trusted the Pilates Method being beneficial for my children. I knew what Pilates could do for Zak, and he had to trust in me. In his high school freshman year, he was the only young man to ever play varsity in the history of Northern Highlands. At one point, I met with his coach because Zak didn't lift weights. The coach demanded, "Zak has to lift weights next year; it's part of team training." I replied, "Zak's not lifting." This was a risky statement because he could have said, "Okay, you know what? Zak won't be playing," but he didn't.

ZAK: So they came to an agreement: if I performed well on the field, then I didn't have to lift weights; if I didn't perform well, then I would start the team's lifting program. When the team was lifting, I ran, rode the bike, did pushups or sit-ups and certain gym exercises on a regular basis. During high school and college my body wasn't fully ready to lift weights because I continued to grow. In high school, my height increased 3-4 inches and I gained 40 pounds. In college, I grew about 1-1½ inches.

KATHI: I look at all the kids who lifted weight so much in high school; they're hurting.

ZAK: Lifting weights, in and of itself, does not result in biomechanically negative outcomes if you supplement it with conditioning that includes stretching and strengthening from internal resistance and working within the weight load of your own body.

KATHI: I spoke with one coach and said, "You have a winning team, and the training must be excellent. But I care about the health and longevity of my son. Of course I want Zak to perform his best, yet I care about him after the game is over; you only care whether the team wins on that field." Some people lose sight of the fact that these young athletes lead lives after their sport. I look at friends of mine who were professional football players; they have had 12-14 surgeries—knees, backs, ankles, hips—and that breaks my heart. I do not want my child to have those serious physical problems or surgeries. Coaches and trainers push athletes to the breaking point. These young athletes don't realize they're all replaceable, and they will be replaced.

ZAK: Switching gears at this point, I would like to mention Dana Santi's Chicago Classical Pilates conferences. For many team members and me, our workout demonstrations at Dana's conferences have been a great opportunity. The first year, team members expected the workout demonstration to include some light stretching; they anticipated enjoying a new experience and feeling good. But when they completed the warm-up, several players asked, "That was just the warm-up? We thought that part of the demo was the whole workout." No one anticipated how vigorous and demanding it would be. By the end of the workout demonstration, they all said, "I feel great. I don't feel beat up like I do after a normal gym or field practice workout. I feel refreshed." They really appreciated the Traditional Pilates workout because it was something new and demanding, which they could apply to football. Sometimes people are afraid of trying something different; I'm fortunate to have friends who are open to learning something new. Every time I brought new kids to Pilates, they really enjoyed it.

I have an Electric Chair/Wunda Chair combination apparatus at school. During the summer, I lived in Chicago, where I interned. When my friends found out, they would say, “Let’s do some Pilates today.” That was really cool for them to make such an effort to try to do it because they really enjoyed it. My sophomore and junior years I frequently trained at Dana’s studio during preseason. My friend Brandon trained there almost every week as well, and the Pilates conditioning definitely showed in his athletic performance. A lot of people don’t understand the importance of strong Traditional Pilates technique. The training is, first and foremost, meant for athletes, boxers, martial artists, and people who vigorously move.

KATHI: Navy Seal workouts were originally based on exercises that include jumping, pushing, and rolling. During the 19th and early 20th centuries, gymnastics and martial arts training were the same. You moved the body; you did pushups, pull-ups, rolled and got yourself up into standing positions. That’s where Joe Pilates’ physical conditioning came from; it was a workout for strong healthy people. But today we have a different conception of gymnastics.

ZAK: I’ve been really fortunate to train with some of the most accomplished teachers: my mom, Jay Grimes, Romana Kryzanowska, Chris Robinson, Dana Santi, Jon Owen, Moses Urbano and others. Because of these intense training experiences, I have a grasp of what Pilates really is. Each teacher has his or her own unique way of approaching the work. My mom may teach one way, yet Moses may have a different style. The important point is that you can learn unique knowledge from each teacher. Everybody can benefit from training in Pilates; it’s definitely helped me become a better athlete.

About Kathryn:

Kathi began her study of The Method in the 1980s. She studied under Romana Kryzanowska and worked with five first generation teachers, striving to carry on their work by teaching and training instructors throughout the world.

Physician Heal Thyself: Corrective Exercise and Chiropractics

By Sandy Shimoda & John Dalcin

The bodies and minds of my students teach me the most...

SANDY: It is widely accepted that the physical attributes of men are different than women. Joe Pilates understood this, and he designed some distinct exercise for men and women that addressed their physical needs. Men are known to have 30-50% more upper body strength that women. Women are known to have greater joint flexibility than men. Body alignment, lung capacity, blood pressure and basal metabolism also differ between the sexes. However, gender is just one factor in determining the best way to teach a client Pilates.

The way I see it, we should view studies about male vs. female with regard to Pilates in the same way we consider tall vs. small, flexible vs. inflexible, and auditory vs. kinesthetic learners. Personally, I don't believe that the separation made by Joe Pilates in addressing male and female physique through exercise were meant to disrespect either gender. In fact, I believe it was quite the opposite. Joe regarded the differences he observed in humans as important indicators in designing a system of exercises that cater to the individual.

As a teacher, it is essential to understand the different bodies and minds that I teach, and to know which exercises will bring the most positive results. Are there exercises for men, opera singers, and elderly people that benefit me? The answer is yes, and I enjoy practicing them on my body so that I can better guide my clients. But those exercises will probably not be the best ones to challenge and positively change the way my body works and feels. Instead, they are tools in my toolbox that I use when they are appropriate.

Helping people to correct the functioning of their body is one of my goals, and training their minds to work in conjunction with their bodies, is another. Finding the best way to communicate Joe Pilates' work to my students is a challenge that I enjoy. In general, I find that men respond better to straightforward instruction with little explanation. But nonetheless each person is unique. Some need more encouragement, lighter touch, help with focus and discipline, or reminders to release tension. The bodies and minds of my students teach me the most about Joe Pilates' great body of work. One fine example is John Dalcin.

John is a stereotypical, masculine man; he is an ex-football player, a jock, an intellectual, a carpenter. He's a man's man. He is also a chiropractor. And although we don't share hobbies or opinions on many subjects, we share a fascination for the human body and the way it moves and functions. Each lesson is a meeting of minds, and his body is our project. John is a medical professional with 35 years' experience ,and his communication style is direct and well-informed. He also has very specific ideas about how a body should move. You can be sure he was challenging from the very first day, and I would be lying if I said he didn't intimidate me at first. But what was important to me was that I wanted to help him; and, of course, I always like a challenge.

JOHN: As a chiropractor, I've seen my share of neuromuscular disorders. But I never imagined one day I would become my own patient. At the age of 55, hip pain became my constant companion. My body hurt like hell, and I could only walk 10 steps before I had to stop and sit down. By the end of a full day treating patients, I was exhausted. At the time, I had heard of Pilates, but I didn't really understand exactly how it benefited the body. From the little I knew, it involved stabilization of the pelvis by working abdominal and gluteal muscles together. I thought it might provide me with some relief, so I began researching Pilates. But I decided to take a novel approach. I actually built a Reformer after finding architectural plans on the Internet. When I finished building the Reformer, I invited my friend Sandy Shimoda to see it. Since she is a Pilates teacher and studio owner, and I valued her expert opinion. Observing her technique, the way she inhabited the movement and worked with the Reformer, it was clear she understood the Pilates system at a profound level; practitioner and apparatus fit together like hand in glove. The visual experience of Sandy's athleticism was like watching a professional jockey at the Kentucky Derby. When she invited me to take lessons to refine my technique, I took her up on the offer, and I was impressed with her teaching and expert knowledge of movement in general.

GETTING STARTED

SANDY: John was an eager and sincere student, but I knew we had a ways to go before he would understand Pilates beyond "stabilization of the pelvis by working abdominal and gluteal muscles together." First of all, I had to get him on Gratz equipment because the Reformer he had so beautifully built defeated Joe's work in so many ways. I knew I couldn't possibly explain how any deviation from Joe's original equipment designs changed the exercises dramatically, and I had no desire to risk insulting John's efforts. Luckily, it only took one lesson for him to feel the difference. The next step was addressing his hip pain. At that time, John's upper body was bent over at the hip and he walked on the toes of one of his feet as a result of chronic hip pain. He was determined to do as much as he could through exercise before succumbing to surgery.

At first John had to do Footwork in 2nd gear because his hips, knees and ankles couldn't bend enough to bring the carriage in without lifting his lower torso off the bed of the Reformer. He was focused on his hips, but I knew he needed to work his whole body. This took hard work, and John grunted and sweated like Jay Grimes describes the men in Joe's New York studio in the '60s. He protested and argued with me at first, but he also gained agility and strength while reducing pain.

HEALER HEAL THYSELF

JOHN: Despite the progress I made with Pilates, my increased strength and flexibility, the inevitable happened. About 2½ years ago, as I was treating a patient in my office, suddenly I felt a "clicking" sensation in my hip. It was the day before I was to embark on a trip to Europe. The following morning I could scarcely walk, but I was determined not to miss the flight, so I just gritted my teeth and bore the pain. When we arrived in Italy, I couldn't walk. Left with no alternative, I quickly checked in to my hotel, where I employed chiropractic methods to alleviate the hip pain. Placing two pillows between my legs, I scissor-squeezed them together for many repetitions. Next morning I woke-up, and to my relief, there was improvement. The trip to Italy was saved. Yet after I returned home, the hip pain and lower body weakness gradually resurfaced. It was challenging to walk steep inclines on mountainsides or near rock cliff formations. I tired easily due to reduced leg strength. In the beginning, pain was a warning signal; but it was the absence of strength that provided clear evidence of hip and leg impairment. Difficulties worsened. Even when I tried to athletically challenge the leg by running or playing golf, energy evaded me. It felt like I was functioning with a dead leg. I could accomplish everyday movements such as standing and walking, but nothing else.

After seeing the MRI images of my hip, it was clear that the best option was a surgical hip replacement. It was a challenging process searching for a highly skilled surgeon whom I could trust. Of course, in my own chiropractic practice I had treated numerous patients with hip replacements. As a result of the surgical technique itself, as well as insufficient muscular rehabilitation, post-surgically their bodies frequently showed evidence of atrophied gluteal muscles, asymmetrical leg length, and a long list of movement restrictions. After researching the work of various hip surgeons, one professional's name kept coming up. So I scheduled an appointment and spoke with him about my concerns. He described the surgical technique for evening leg length; he would remove the damaged part of my hip without cutting any muscle; and he anticipated that I wouldn't have any movement restrictions. "That sounds great," I said, "and I know the perfect professional to guide me through post-surgical, corrective exercise." At that time, I had been studying with Sandy for a while, so I had an understanding of Pilates. Within one week after the hip surgery, I resumed training with her. As a result, I challenge anyone to tell me which hip was replaced. The reality is that I'm in better shape now at age 61 than at 54. I can do anything.

PILATES AND CHIROPRACTIC CARE

SANDY: Using Pilates to address a problem that had ailed John for nearly a decade made a believer out of him—so much so that he wanted his patients to share in the benefits of doing Pilates. He asked me where he could get certified to become a teacher. But after some discussion, he realized that he was not interested in changing careers, and at 61 he didn't need another certification. To be honest, I don't think he would have endured a certification program. John is a passionate healer and knows the body far beyond what is required to be a Pilates teacher. After a few years of studying with me he already had such a sophisticated grasp of Joe's work, and was articulate in the way he described it, so I agreed to take him on as an apprentice so as to help him understand the system as a whole. Each week after he did his Reformer or Mat workout, I took him through the main exercises on each piece of equipment. He was like a kid in a playground. I could see his mind and body understanding the distinct value of each piece of equipment. So much so that he began building other pieces of apparatus at his office: ladder barrel, big chair, even a Cadillac. He would work his body with such joy, spontaneously grinning as he found new ways to move through the stiffness in his body. In truth, there was no stopping him. With or without my help, John was going to find a way to deliver Joe's work to his clients as a complement to chiropractic care.

JOHN: In my chiropractic office, patients regularly utilize Pilates apparatus for neuromuscular retraining—what Joe Pilates called "corrective exercise"—to reduce challenging symptoms and gain strength, flexibility, coordination, and responsiveness. Deterioration of the low back usually starts at L5/S1; this area corresponds to the lower abdominal region in the coronal, frontal plane. Without sufficient abdominal articulation-strength, which enables vertebral column sequencing, the human torso tends to hinge "in one piece" from hip joints to complete various physical actions. This results in overuse of the iliopsoas muscle and an increased probability of developing back pain symptoms. Traditional Pilates technique reverses this problem by coordinating gluteal muscle work and upwardly lifting abdominals to facilitate elongation of back muscles, which all provide support for optimal functioning of the L4-L5 area. Pilates provides a system for regaining normal-range, spine/hip mobility; vertebral sequencing; and improved carriage of the entire skeleton as people age. Although the age clock cannot be reversed, individuals can certainly gain strength, flexibility, and control of muscle groups associated with The Center. In turn, daily movements and skilled sports are optimized. To develop biomechanical health, it is key to initiate abdominal muscles before spinal muscles to sequentially bend the spine.

SANDY: John is not the first medical professional to see the benefits of Pilates for rehabilitation and conditioning of the body. But he understands that there is no comparison between practicing Pilates as a system of exercise, and using a few exercises to prepare a client for spinal adjustment or to help them understand how to retrain specific patterns of movement. John is not a Pilates teacher, but he employs some of its principles to serve his clients.

JOHN: Pilates stands on its own as a valid mental and physical conditioning technique when taught by a quality professional with good insight. In my chiropractic medical practice, I incorporate certain Pilates exercises using the Reformer and Cadillac, enabling clients to achieve a different awareness or improved coordination in lower back, knee, hip, or shoulder rehabilitation. There's no difference in my approach, whether I'm working with a man or a woman. People are people. They're interested in healing and thriving. My goals are to alleviate pain and facilitate improved structure, posture, and alignment. In my practice, I use a combination of disciplines: chiropractics, physical therapy, and Pilates. Much of my knowledge comes from training sessions with Sandy. She is an extraordinary teacher; each lesson has different combinations of exercises, and I can see the crossover with all of them. Because of my medical training and the way my mind naturally works, I see how sequences of exercises relate within and between one another on different studio apparatus. You can practice a series of exercises on the Cadillac that resemble exercises on the Reformer so The Work is qualitatively different because of utilizing another apparatus with distinct dimensions, which change your base of support, center of gravity, skeletal angle, and balance.

Practicing any physical activity requires energy. As human beings, we can get tired, even exhausted with various responsibilities and aspirations. This situation can affect workout frequency. For me, the key is to vary the duration as well as the exercises in the Pilates system. On Saturdays, I have my lesson with Sandy. During weekdays I've been practicing, deepening my understanding and accomplishing exercises on my own. Essentially, I have been discovering The Method for myself while studying with a great teacher. As a result, I'm more proficient and self-sufficient, which Sandy said Joe Pilates wanted for his students.

SANDY: In addition to what he does in his chiropractic office, I have challenged John beyond his daily application of Pilates. He has taken students through complete Mat and Reformer workouts, and each student has walked away with a new understanding of how to use Pilates for specific challenges in their bodies. John's personal progress is a testament to his belief in Joe's work, an intellectual and physical understanding of Pilates principles, and a willingness to use his body to learn.

JOHN'S PROCESS

JOHN: First and foremost, I have total respect for and trust in Sandy. If she says, "You're not stretching enough through your legs while lifting from your Center," either we'll work on improving the movement or change to another exercise, depending upon which choice seems more beneficial. I have complete confidence in her insights, observations, and instructions, which deepen my understanding of the work, and I listen and strive to accomplish both the intention and action of each exercise. After all, I'm a 61-year-old guy. I work as hard as I can to achieve these exercises, and I'm lacking in many respects. I understand what Sandy wants me to accomplish as far as muscular action: how to engage The Center, direct the energy, and create the shape of the exercise. On a scale from 1-10 with 10, being the best, maybe I'll achieve between 3-4 or 6-7. I'm not going to be a 10. That's okay; I just don't have it anymore. What's important is that Pilates definitely stopped "the backslide," of my body's health and vitality. It has already added years of quality living to my life. For that, I am very grateful. Pilates activates the body-brain connection. If you practice exercises with precision and competency, you become more mentally awake; that's why Joe Pilates described his work as physical and mental conditioning. You don't gain anything by practicing Pilates ineffectively or inefficiently. Not that achieving perfection is the goal, but one should always aim toward progress. Even though you might not be technically proficient, you can still improve. When you bring all the elements together, you'll find yourself thinking, *Okay, that's how the exercise should feel; that's what athletic skill, good concentration, and timing can be.*

When I look at some people working out, it's clear they have superior flexibility and precision. Some of the individuals are athletes and some are dancers. They look skillfully artistic. When I started Pilates six years ago, I could see the striking contrast between their work and mine. Yet there's really no comparison. In this system of body conditioning, there's no competition except with yourself and Joe's method. Have you ever seen archival pictures of the nonathletic people whom Joe Pilates trained in his original studio? I'm more like them. When I began training with Sandy, I was exercising my body with a non-Pilates approach. That's because most men of every age are socialized with different kinds of body awareness compared to women. So, when men try Pilates, they start with a sports mentality and must evolve into ways of knowing associated with Pilates; in short, it's a different mind-set. In my case, I'm no longer trying to muscle through exercises anymore; I'm connecting and distributing fluid strength. And I have improved balance and coordinated reaction time. Say I am working on a house project, but I'm standing on a ladder when I have to reach down for the socket wrench. Because of Pilates, my body is more under the control of my mind; therefore, I can accomplish the movement with confidence and ease. The same is true of athletic activity as well as daily activity. Just standing from a sitting position, then walking to the water cooler is an important daily accomplishment. Consider the simple acts of walking up stairs, moving boxes, planting the garden, cleaning the shower, sitting in your car, even teaching Pilates!

NOT BETTER, NOT WORSE, JUST APPROPRIATE

SANDY: With John as an example, we can evaluate our ideas around men in Pilates. Is John the student he is because he is a man? How was his process affected by the fact that he is a chiropractor? What part did pain play in the way he learned? As a teacher, it is my job to take all of these elements into consideration when I teach John. One thing that has helped my teaching is to see the exercises objectively. There is no exercise that is better or worse, just more appropriate. John's memory of one important lesson is a great illustration of that.

JOHN: A week after my hip surgery, I walked through the front door of Vintage Pilates with a cane. When the lesson was over, I carried my cane as I walked out of the studio! Sandy introduced me to an apparatus called the Foot Corrector. Afterwards, I could feel my body's alignment through the entire skeletal chain. When I train in Pilates, my muscles work through my feet, connecting through my knees and awakening the entire body above into hips, waist, chest, shoulders, neck, and crown of the head. The body falls into its own "plum line" of verticality and stabilization by lifting and extending in axial elongation. By practicing Pilates, you stabilize your body for movement by extending inward and upward, by making your body vertically longer rather than sinking lower, compressing muscles and joints and dragging your body down. Instead of plodding along like a worn-out plow horse, you become a thoroughbred racehorse.

SANDY: I am grateful to John for teaching me through his enthusiasm, intelligence, and love for everything he does. His voice speaks volumes about the significance of Pilates as a man, a medical professional, an athlete, and an outstanding human being. His work in the studio has helped me to discover what is both challenging and beautiful about the differences in the ways individuals move and think.

About Sandy:

Sandy Shimoda has been teaching movement since the 1980s and was introduced to Pilates in 1994. She has been a private student of Jay Grimes since 2004 and opened Vintage Pilates with the hope of providing a place for students to access the wealth of understanding that Jay has to offer. Sandy has been a demonstrator on GAIAM and Classical Pilates videos and has been featured in Pilates Style and in Pilatesglossy.com.

How Can Pilates Combat Slouching & Increase Athletic Longevity in Men?

By Karen Courtland Kelly

...There is no age restriction because the exercises are for everyone.

Modern man is a casualty of today's technological revolution. Our days are spent slouched over the computer, the tablet, or cell phone, engrossed in the latest texts or tweets. More sedentary than previous generations, men suffer from its effects with poor posture. But the Pilates Method of Body Conditioning addresses this problem. Pilates corrects slouching by efficiently targeting the core (the Pilates Powerhouse), simultaneously lengthening the body's extremities. This combination of factors develops a more athletic body, increases athletic longevity, and enhances the quality of life. It improves posture, over-all health, coordination, flexibility, and efficient movement. The result is a more energized body and a sense of well-being. Long before our technological revolution, Joseph Pilates recognized that exercise is critical for everyone, calling for a "Return to Life."

The effectiveness of the Pilates Method lies in the inextricable relationship between the apparatus and the six Pilates principles:

- Concentration
- Control
- Centering
- Breath
- Precision
- Flow of movement

These principles apply to all sports, as well as daily life. Concentration facilitates control, enabling movement to come from the center. Through breath and precision of movement, the capacity to flow in and out of the exercises changes the quality of movement. Use of the six principles facilitates awareness of correct posture. Whether sitting, walking, or playing sports, one must combat slouching in order to maintain proper postural alignment. And slouching, as well as obesity, is a big problem today, even in young people. It is critical for men to avoid slouching if they wish to maintain health, improve appearance, and enjoy athletic endeavors for many more years.

As a female Pilates teacher, I've learned a great deal over the years from my husband, Patrick, who is an Olympic speed skater and former McGill hockey player. He is a trained mechanical engineer, so he approaches Pilates much like I do; I envision Joseph Pilates developing his apparatus in the same way that Leonardo Davinci approached his canvas or Michelangelo created a sculpture. Pilates invented the apparatus visualizing the exercises and the goals he wished to achieve with the body. Not every exercise is for every body.

Patrick has deepened my understanding of the difference in the physical and emotional makeup of men and women. And this insight has changed the way I teach men; I give them more breathing room during a Pilates session, even if that man happens to be my husband. Patrick strives for exceptional technique and knows what he needs to accomplish, so I just refine The Work, but I don't tinker with what isn't broken. Too many corrections can be unwelcome, so it is important to back off and let men discover The Work.

Neither Patrick nor I knew anything about Pilates until later in our athletic careers. We both competed in the 1994 Winter Olympic Games in Lillehammer, Norway. I participated in the pairs event with my skating partner, Todd Reynolds; and Patrick competed in the 500, 1,000, and 1,500 meter speed skating races. Although neither of us came home with Olympic medals, we did find each other, meeting in the cafeteria at the Olympic Village.

During our athletic careers, we both experienced our share of ups and downs. Patrick broke a leg in seven places and was told he would never walk normally again, let alone skate at the Olympics. I endured a seven-year career slump. These setbacks taught us the meaning of perseverance, the necessity of forging ahead before one's life changes course. Learning how to work through adversity and make responsible decisions grounded us, made us appreciate the gifts we were given.

After the Olympics, we had to transition our lives, as well as our bodies. As figure skaters, Todd and I trained and executed figure eights regularly, but we never understood how to work both sides of the body evenly. Unlike the dancer's basic ballet barre, designed to train the body symmetrically, we developed muscle imbalances, resulting in overuse injuries. During our Olympic days, our coaches didn't focus on developing body symmetry, and as athletes, we failed to recognize the need. Given the gift of athleticism, we were cursed with high pain tolerance and, working through injuries just exacerbated them. Unfortunately, at that time we didn't know about the benefits of the Pilates Method of Body Conditioning.

Rehabilitating overuse injuries and muscle imbalances takes a lot of work, but the biggest challenge is finding the correct treatment protocol and the best practitioner to address the issue. Suffering from overuse injuries after The Games, luckily I found Pilates. I began working with a gifted physical therapist, Linda Tremain, who worked on the imbalances everywhere, from every part of my foot to the top of my head. Linda encouraged me to explore Pilates training in addition to physical therapy, recommending Juanita Lopez at the Pilates Studio in Evanston, Illinois. Linda's knowledge and kindness set me on the pathway to healing. She and many other phenomenal people with whom I worked are the reason why I am healthier today than when I competed in the Olympics. Eventually, Patrick's and my life took us back East, and I continued my Pilates training in New York City with Romana and Sari at Drago's Gym from 1996-2001.

During my journey, I taught my husband Pilates. As student and teacher, we acquired functional knowledge through the Pilates Method. It's really how you use it and how you pass it on. Patrick knows how to take just five minutes a day to make a difference in a specific part of his body. Although this takes time to learn, the functionality of the Pilates Method is worth the learning curve.

Patrick likes the creativity of Pilates. It isn't a chore for him; he uses it to enhance his life. Most of his work is on the Reformer, executing exercises that his body needs. In particular, he strengthens his powerhouse, completing an abbreviated Reformer with advanced arm/shoulder exercises crucial for his hockey playing. He also enjoys Rolling Like a Ball.

Patrick understands that it is important to use the Pilates apparatus to help the body overcome its physical and/or mental limitations. Creativity is a key aspect of The Work; just look at how creative Joseph

Pilates was, inventing a variety of apparatus and a range of mat exercises. But it is important to have fun with all the apparatus and mat exercises best suited for your body

Always keep a sense of humor! Use your gifts to bring out the best in each client instead of imposing limitations. I've worked with so many people on so many different levels, from professional athletes to novices to injured clients who work one step at a time. Despite their level of expertise and fitness, they all face impediments to their progress. It is important not to limit them, but to determine how to help them overcome any mental, physical, or emotional sticking points. Just ask yourself, "How is that person blocked? Is he thinking about something in the wrong way or is he worried about something?" In athletics, focusing on a negative thought blocks the pathway to the goal.

Ask the client, "Are you comfortable with this? How are you feeling?" Then adjust the movement accordingly, remembering that each client is a complete individual with his own life experiences that affect him. Clients should feel free and enjoy doing The Work, learning it in a way that enables them to process and enjoy it. Reminding a man to keep his sense of humor is critical to the learning process. Try to be fluid in how you work with each person because it's not about the teacher. The teacher should help the client accomplish the movement, encouraging him:

- To relax and try to be less self-conscious/critical about learning something new.
- To enjoy the process of learning; it is humbling.
- Not to feel bad if he can't execute a Pilates exercise right away (this is very important).
- To communicate right away if something doesn't feel right during an exercise.
- To feel emotionally supported and encouraged to learn Pilates.
- To communicate his insights and questions.

It is important to recognize when something isn't working. If a client is not comfortable with a particular movement, even if it would be good for him, move on. It is fine to say, "We don't have to do that," or "Let's come back to that later." Remind him, "It's a work in progress," and finish the session praising him for a job well done. When he returns the following week, he will look forward to his lesson.

Everybody learns in different ways with different timetables and there are so many exercises available that it is important not to get stuck in the same box for all clients. Certainly there is the foundation and each client should learn good Pilates technique. But sometimes it is necessary to modify the workout based on a client's emotional and/or physical responses. Do so in a gentle and efficient way, and come back to the challenging exercise later. When the mind and body are ready, the execution is easy. And the client is happy.

Remember:

- Learning takes time.
- It is best not to rush the whole process; absorb the work and learn something about your body in each session.
- Sometimes it's about slowing down and taking the time to be attentive.

Learning Pilates can be overwhelming, so it is critical to avoid embarrassment as clients navigate the learning curve. In order to learn how to move from The Center with precision, one needs to be open to corrections. But it is difficult to know how a particular client will react to the instruction. In a group class, I verbally cue the correction without singling anyone out. It becomes a general instruction for all participants.

Demonstrating the correction seems to work well. I might suggest, "Pay attention to the foot," as I show the proper way to move. Then the client makes the adjustment without feeling embarrassed in front of the class. Not everyone has a dance or athletic background in which constant correction is simply a part of training, "Fix this. Fix that. Your foot is rolling in. Your knees are not aligned." The athlete understands that his trainer has good intentions, preparing him for completion. It is not as easy for a Pilates client to understand that his trainer simply wants him to achieve his best. So it is incumbent on the teacher to develop trust by correcting in such a way that the client feels comfortable and confident.

Patrick has taught me that sometimes a teacher needs to step back when giving a correction, introducing the exercise but giving the client space to learn. Men need time and space to learn and absorb the movement in their own way. When clients feel less self-conscious, they feel better about the correction or the exercise. So making someone comfortable learning The Work is absolutely critical. This way clients stay with Pilates for life.

And Pilates, like every sport or art, should be a lifelong adventure, a discipline one loves. Of course, life sometimes gets in the way. People's schedules change, family and work make demands on us. But by making clients feel welcome, they return when circumstances change. They remember, "Pilates makes me feel better."

That is because Pilates helps men's bodies become more intelligent! But this takes time. So it is imperative to engage men, draw them in to The Work. When a man begins to study Pilates, ask him about himself, how he is feeling, and what brought him to Pilates. Often men come to Pilates because they know it's good for them, but they don't necessarily want to be there. Generate interest by teaching them tidbits about Joseph Pilates, explaining how he invented apparatus to help himself become a better athlete.

Generally it's good to center the body on the Reformer first. Since not all men are comfortable in Pilates stance, sometimes I start athletes in parallel. Get them moving in good alignment and don't make them feel that you're nitpicking. Focus on using the Powerhouse, lengthening the back, and stretching out the legs. This is important, especially if men have office jobs. Remaining in a seated position for long periods of time tightens hamstrings and hip flexors, often causing back pain. Elongating the legs alleviates pressure on the spine and improves posture. Move on to The Hundred, which is an exercise men often dislike, as it makes them feel awkward. Find the optimal position for that particular man, encourage him to activate the core, and keep corrections to a minimum.

While men should learn the Reformer, it is important to use other apparatus as well, focusing on the client's specific needs. Many men are stiff, but the Roll-Back opens up the back, lengthens the spine, and strengthens the Powerhouse. This lack of flexibility affects posture and, as we know from Joseph Pilates, a person is only as young as his spine.

Reinforce the notion that Pilates combats slouching, improving posture by using the Powerhouse to lengthen the spine. I explain that, "Gravity pushes the human body down and out, but Pilates pulls us in and up." Once men have this focus, challenge them in a way that's safe and healthy, building their Powerhouse. Be attentive to their specific needs: tight shoulders, back, chest, hamstrings, calves or quads; flat feet; and mental/emotional state. The psychological aspect is just as important as physicality. Attending to both results in a happy client who feels so much better when he leaves than when he came in.

A teacher knows she has connected with a client when he recognizes the effect of an exercise on his body, "You know, I think we should do that exercise we tried last week. I think I need that one today." He is thinking, feeling, and understanding The Work on a deeper level.

Tips for working with a man who has worked behind a desk for 30 years, but still wants to play golf and tennis like he did in his youth!

Men can be impatient, failing to understand why they lack the agility and flexibility they possessed in their younger years. They are incredulous at their lackluster tennis game or their inability to dash to court after sitting behind a desk for five hours. They never needed to warmup before nine holes of golf. I explain that age has something to do with it, but not everything. If the Powerhouse isn't working, everything in the body goes, whether young or old. The key is to train the core. It might take a little more time to come back the older one gets, but even young people today have poor posture, lack of flexibility, and diminished strength. Just look around you. It is critical that we pass on the love and the joy of movement.

Tips on training athletic men!

Athletes are so much fun to work with. I've taught professional tennis players, golfers, and ironman competitors, as well as skaters and even martial artists who have achieved black belts. The first issue I address is the perception men often have that only women do Pilates. They are surprised to learn that a man actually invented Pilates, but are often skeptical of the ability to experience a vigorous workout. So I give them a challenging Pilates session.

When a teacher encourages good technique and good alignment, the client can really experience the benefits of working on the Reformer, progressing at his own rate. It is a real joy to guide super athletes such as martial artists to an advanced level. This is the perfect opportunity to use the Reformer in all its capacity, from the basic work to the Rowing series, Snake and Twist, and the Splits.

Challenge clients on all the apparatus so they benefit from the entire method: Pull-Ups, Chin-Ups, supine and standing Arm Springs. Given the chosen sport, what does that particular body need? Skaters develop better leg alignment with Single Leg Squats on the Cadillac, enabling them to better execute Shoot the Duck, a similar movement on the ice.

When awareness happens, seize the moment. One client, a hypermobile tennis pro, recognized his weakness during a Reformer workout; he actually felt how he wasn't stabilizing his Center enough. I explained, "The Reformer is teaching you what you need to know so you can be a better professional tennis player and teacher." Instead of feeling inadequate, this concept was critical in his learning process. I explained, "Pilates always finds your weakness. That's the function of the apparatus and why Pilates is so effective! It leads you to recognition, and when the correct exercises are selected, it allows you to strengthen the area safely." The Method has something for everyone.

Every day the body feels different, depending on diet, sleep, and what's going on in one's life. So take Pilates as constructive feedback. The apparatus communicates with you. And the joy of the communication between the body and the apparatus is dynamic, expressing what it needs through feedback from the springs on the apparatus.

This is especially true for an athlete with an injury or weakness. Pay attention when the badminton or tennis player with previous injuries confesses, "My shoulder is hurting." It may be important to avoid certain exercises, selecting those that build the weak area. Work around what he needs, so he is in his body. It takes work to get it right. But the more diversely the body is trained, the more prepared it is for any sport.

Tips on working with men making a comeback!

Men returning to exercise after a hiatus due to injury or the demands of life suffer the effects of lack of exercise and improper technique. This client has to build up his body slowly and the teacher must encourage him to appreciate that dynamic wisely. Instead of feeling stressed or inadequate, embrace the situation, viewing this as an opportunity to improve. Rebuild the body with basic Reformer, remembering that in any sport performing the basics well is difficult. Mastering the basic work is critical for success. Even teachers and advanced students don't need to do the advanced work every time. Revisiting the foundation improves the advanced workout. Practice basic Reformer; do some electric chair, some Wunda chair, and some Mat exercises. Feel good, re-center, use The Method and the beauty of the basics, and do them well. Then build back up to the advanced work. Practice flow.

Flow is a more important concept than some might think. In the Pilates system, practitioners flow from one exercise to the next. But flow exists in all fitness modalities, sports, and physical activities. There are ebbs and flows, peaks and valleys. An athlete peaks and then he loses that competitive edge. The injured athlete, who resumes training after a temporary interruption, experiences the ebb and flow of a sports career. And there is the flow of life within the Pilates work, enabling one to reap the benefits of The Work without feeling bad. With experience, it is possible to achieve a new understanding of flow, "I used to do the advanced work, but right now I'm not capable of executing those moves; still, I know I can rebuild with the basics."

To reinforce the benefits of The Method, practice Pilates in surprising places! I teach clients how to utilize Pilates just about anywhere, even standing in line at the grocery store. Place feet in Pilates stance, pull the belly button in, and draw the shoulders down. Make sure the back is lengthened and hips are under. Use your Powerhouse just standing there. To correct slouching, work the internal symmetry and the mind. Concentrate on being centered in the midst of our chaotic world. Instead of seething over the long line ahead of you, use the time to do something productive and helpful. Take Pilates out of the studio and put it into your life. Use it to mentally or physically accomplish any task. That is when The Work becomes the most relevant and useful.

Guide clients to move from being attentive to being intelligent with their bodies! This is an issue of quality versus quantity. The oft repeated mantra, "Practice makes perfect," is not necessarily true. Perfect practice leads to more perfect movement. A few movements, executed with concentration and control, are more effective than many repetitions performed sloppily. When an exercise seems impossible, just go with the flow, modifying the workout as necessary.

If a client is on autopilot, lacking concentration, suggest, "Maybe, we should get out of the routine, change it up a bit." There are so many pieces of apparatus available. Dust off the Foot Corrector and Spine Corrector to improve posture! The Foot Corrector develops small neurological and muscular patterns from the foot through the top of the head. In Pilates it is the minute details that make a big difference. And Joseph Pilates knew how important it is to strengthen the feet, because a stronger base leads to better posture.

Even after 20 years of practice, one can still have moments of insight. I've had some clients who were not comfortable doing the Short Box on the Reformer, critical to improve posture. I tried my best to work around it. One day, working out at the studio by myself, I began to play on the Spine Corrector. A moment of insight occurred as I glanced at the Tower mat. At the end of the mat there is a foot strap for the Roll-Up. "Ah-ha, I'm going to take the Spine Corrector, put it at the end of the mat, and use the strap like I'm sitting up on the Reformer for Short Box." I thought, *Well, I've never seen it, but it sure feels good.* I believe that Romana, Sari, and Joseph Pilates would be comfortable with this because I modified The Work in a safe, efficient way for someone who is not comfortable executing the move on the Reformer. I just knew my client would feel the Spine Corrector support his back.

So the next time he came to the studio, I said, "I have a surprise for you. We're going to try something new today." I placed his feet under the strap, and made sure the Spine Corrector was far enough back for his legs, knees not too locked, not too bent. As I began teaching the Short Box series on the Spine Corrector, suddenly he was able to accomplish the exercises, strengthening his Powerhouse. Now he enjoys doing The Tree. With pillows under his head, he can open his chest. Able to go all the way back and hold the stretch, he gets the benefit from The Tree in a safe way. And he is better able to combat slouching. As a teacher, I'm not stressed; and as a student, he's happy. Just a little creativity enabled him to accomplish an otherwise impossible exercise.

But my work doesn't end here. I do my part in this battle for better posture wherever I am, urging anyone and everyone, "Please put the computer down. If you've been at the desk a long time, stand for Chest Expansion and then do Double Leg Kicks from the Mat exercises. It's one of the greatest anti-slouching exercises ever. It strengthens your powerhouse, stretches your quads, opens the chest, and straightens the whole spine from leaning forward." As teachers, we must remember that Pilates is not just a workout; it is a way of life!

---

[1] Pilates, Joseph H. Return to Life. Presentation Dynamics, Incline Village, NV. (2000), p.1.

About Karen:

Karen Courtland Kelly is a U.S. Olympian who loves to promote skating and Pilates to all for sport, health, and socializing. She is a professional performer, trained teacher, motivational speaker, and spokesperson who is passionate about academics and athletics.

Pilates Fitness Over 50

By José Antonio Lopez & Marta Cristina Diaz Velasco

...There is no age restriction because the exercises are for everyone.

JOSÉ: My wife, Andrea Aburto, and I started training with Marta Christina Diaz Velasco about a year ago. Since convenience is important, we searched for a Traditional Pilates studio near our house. Believe me, it's not easy to find excellent instruction in the real Pilates Method, so we felt fortunate to find True Pilates Chile, just ten minutes from us. Her teaching style and fully-equipped studio impressed us. At the time, we had recently returned from New Zealand, where we trained with a Pilates teacher who was nowhere near Marta's caliber. Marta finds a way to help us achieve important fitness conditioning goals and makes each lesson enjoyable with a wide variety of exercises. The work is mentally challenging and interesting, and the exercise routine varies every time; that's what makes the whole difference.

MARTA: Thank you, José. My teaching style is a direct result of working with Romana at True Pilates and Inelia in Sao Paulo. Romana taught me about flow, dynamic movement. She often said, "Pilates is poetry in motion. It is a science of the body and an art form." In contrast, Inelia tends to be very technical in her teaching, so it takes a long time for students to understand it's okay to move with energy and fluidity.

JOSÉ: I first observed Pilates at Drago's Gym in New York City. At the time, someone I knew who was studying Pilates suggested, "Why don't you look at the studio and take a lesson?" I only visited the studio twice, but when I saw people working out, I had the sense of Pilates being very different compared to body conditioning taught in regular gyms or health clubs; in part because the exercises and equipment are so different, and in part because people seemed to truly enjoy themselves! Everyone in the studio was flexible! No one had a big body or overdeveloped muscles. Their movements were natural, strong, fluid and beautiful. I immediately thought, *Ah, this is what I would like to* *do; this is the way I would like my mind and body to be.* The Pilates system has so many different exercises, which makes The Work creative and interesting. When I came to study with Marta, I had the same sense of her studio and teaching as I did at Drago's.

The primary change I experienced in my body is improved flexibility. At first I didn't even realize my flexibility was increasing. Yet now I can accomplish many physical activities that I couldn't imagine a year ago. This makes me feel really good. Sometimes Marta would say, "I'm impressed with how much you've improved since starting Pilates." Since I started practicing Pilates, my back problems have virtually disappeared. The positive comments by other people, too, reflect the benefits of Pilates training; I hear compliments from others about my health, strength, energy, and vitality. My health is important to me, especially now that I'm a 60-year-old, first-time father of a 2-year-old boy, Mateo! This is exciting and challenging at the same time. I'm always picking up Mateo, playing with him, and taking care of him, just like fathers who are much younger than I; and it's because of Pilates! What a gift to be strong, flexible, and vigorous at my age! Periodically when I encounter former schoolmates, they ask, "How do you stay in such good physical shape and participate in so many athletic activities?" Although some friends know I study Pilates, most just think, *You look fit and healthy.*

During a recent road trip, I drove my car for 24 hours over the course of 2 days. We stopped for a rest along the way, deciding to walk through the hills for another 2-3 hours before arriving back home. I didn't feel fatigued, proof that individuals my age can condition their bodies and minds just like someone far younger. Yet, it's not just any kind of conditioning; it's Traditional Pilates. The secret is that Pilates combines particular kinds of strengthening and stretching using your own body weight. Because of Pilates I can function physically at peak levels all day. On any given day, I wake up early in the morning, work in the garden, shower with Mateo, and perform many more chores, such as repairing the fireplace chimney or trimming the hedges around the house.

MARTA: José is a delightful student; he enjoys coming to lessons, loves The Work, and appreciates the way in which Pilates educates his body. That makes a real difference. When José first came to my studio, he was so inflexible, he could not touch his toes. He also had significant lumbar pain and stress. Now he is symptom-free with increased flexibility and physical health achieved through Pilates. José can reach, stretch, twist, bend, and extend much farther in biomechanically correct ways. Remember that Joe Pilates described his method as "corrective exercise." José has indeed reaped the benefits of corrective exercise!

JOSÉ: When I first started Pilates training, I had to learn what Marta meant when she used particular technical terms. When you don't understand the words, you don't know what to do; it's like learning a language, a language of movement. Once you comprehend the meaning, then you understand how to move. To this end, it's often helpful if the instructor uses common phrases instead of technical terms; referring to the scapula or shoulder blades as "wings" makes the intention clearer to the client.

I truly enjoy being in the studio, taking lessons with Marta. Although we share laughs, I always maintain focus because correct movement requires constant intelligent choices. Attention must be paid to the balance between placement, alignment, and flowing movement. Traditional Pilates is Traditional Pilates. Despite this fact, there are different approaches between well-trained teachers. Instructors trained by Inelia focus on technically correct movement. Students who trained with Romana focus on form as well, but they emphasize flowing movement, rhythm, and dynamics; it's an athletic art form.

Marta tells me that the foundation of Joe Pilates' work includes the spirit, as well as mental and physical conditioning. Of course, this is a complex area of human experience to explore. However, for me, this unity in the traditional Pilates technique complements my studies in Buddhism. The ways in which I think and feel foster a union of effective concentration, continuous and rewarding spiritual work. When I organize projects, coordinate events, or achieve goals in my professional work or personal life, my friends and colleagues seem appreciative. Why? Because I achieve optimal levels of "the art of control" in my daily life. In contrast, when people feel stressed or distracted, they are unable to find balance personally or professionally. My studies in traditional Pilates cultivate mental and spiritual presence, or "conditioning," as Joe Pilates described it, filling a reservoir with overall intelligence and skill-based action. This translates to improved performance in the world of work. Although I never sought the position of general manager in my profession, it was offered to me because I have good organizational skills, enhanced by Pilates and Buddhism. These physical and mental disciplines contribute to my creativity and improve my overall health. Renewed energy, strength, insight, consciousness, flexibility, and alertness give me an advantage.

MARTA: The body is a beautiful and spectacular machine that is very wise if you cultivate the proper attention and distribute the right amount of energy. Using right intention while working on traditional apparatus teaches you how to direct your energy and awareness.

JOSÉ: Marta is absolutely right. The body is full of energy, but it's the way you use your body that blocks energy or facilitates flowing movement. As time progresses, body and mind harmonize by channeling the mind through coordinated movement. Exercises become more fluid; the body becomes more flexible. Then you feel energy release and support new movements, which, in turn, develop increased awareness, further improving technique. When energy is stuck in your body, there is more potential for strain or injury. And having the right equipment is important; it must be classical. I've traveled quite a bit and taken lessons with various teachers who have different equipment. Although I don't understand the mechanics, my body feels the difference.

MARTA: Energy can flow through your body in a much more perfect way when you're correctly aligned, when you have good coordination, and when you're not putting stress in your joints, muscles, bones, or nervous system. As your physical health improves, you develop improved emotional health and lightheartedness. So keep moving, keep making progress, freeing yourself to attain optimal health and well-being. In these ways, you have more energy. You can feel it! Previously, José had serious lumbar pain. I learned an important lesson from Romana when I had similar, painful symptoms. She recommended that I use the Spine Corrector, which was very helpful. Romana was brilliant; instinctively she knew what students could accomplish before they realized their own capabilities. In turn, I do my best to assess each student's capacity to transform their limitations through the corrective exercise method of Contrology.

JOSÉ: I practice meditation. And Pilates is a combination of physical, spiritual, and mental work, which, when combined, constitute meditation in motion. The union of physical, spiritual, and mental in traditional Pilates is transformative; the system allows us to transcend problems, overcome limitations, and realize our full potential. When I train with Marta, I'm "in the moment," so to speak. My concentration is pure. These qualities are also central aims of Buddhism; to be fully in the present in each moment. During each lesson with Marta, there's nothing in my mind except what Marta is teaching, what I'm experiencing and the ways in which my body, mind, and spirit are evolving in complementary ways. This is key. Because the human mind seeks intensity and equilibrium, the complexity of Pilates keeps me engaged.

MARTA: The Work of Traditional Pilates promotes health and well-being; Joe Pilates' unique system of mental and physical conditioning enables the body and mind to realize their full intelligence, improving over time. Suddenly, you feel more passionate about life! Teachers and students see the value in The Work, especially in their daily lives, and, therefore, they reap extraordinary rewards. That's why my students are eager to quickly return after each holiday; they're all here the first week because they need the Pilates in their bodies. As José notes, energy is important; it's the basis of vitality. We also need energy to fuel the muscles. If you lack energy, you don't want to move your body. By investing energy in your workout, you receive an abundant return of energy for your daily life.

JOSÉ: People who know that I train with Marta inquire, "Why are you doing Pilates?" They ask because in Latin America there's a macho mentality, a male code of behavior embracing strength, force, dominance, and financial success. Symbolically, they all go together. Yet Pilates is advertised and perceived as women's exercise. It is misunderstood as a feminine activity, which is not physically demanding enough for men. Most men believe you have to train muscles with heavy weights and work them to fatigue. But Joe Pilates understood that building too much muscle mass slows down muscle reaction time in sports, boxing, and martial arts. He didn't believe in lifting heavy weights and developing bulky muscles. He advocated using your own body weight to develop uniform muscular development. When other men see the results of Pilates in my body, my increased energy capacity, they announce, "I want to try Pilates." For excellent reasons, I think there is big potential for more men to train in the classical system. The development of Pilates for men parallels other social changes. In

Chile, more men are learning the art of cooking, more men are studying yoga, and more men are simply getting more physical exercise in order to stay healthy.

Here's my advice to all men: take a good look at the photos of Joe Pilates demonstrating his system of body conditioning. He was a serious German tough guy, a boxer and athlete. He created a strong method of exercise that enhances every aspect of your life. I know first-hand. My training with Marta Christina De Velasco enables me to function at maximum performance every day in every endeavor. There is no age restriction because the exercises are for everyone. Students can progress at their own pace, and lessons are individualized. Pilates benefits every body!

About Marta:

Marta is the owner and director of True Pilates Chile in Santiago de Chile. Marta is passionate about preserving Joe Pilates' traditional system of body conditioning, and sharing her knowledge, with students as well as teachers from around the world. Marta completed her education and training with master teacher Romana Kryzanowska in New York, NY.

Marta has also trained with Sari Mejia Santo, Jerome Weinberg, Cynthia Shipley, Pamela Pardi, Javier Perez Pont, Esperanza Aparicio, Chacha Guerrero, Francisca Molina, Kathi Ross-Nash, Dorothee VanderWalle, Alycea Ungaro, Inelia García and Peter Fiasca.

Stretch, Strength, and Control

By Martin Spencker & Amanda Diatta

...The Method deftly addressed my misalignment and muscle imbalances...

When I tell male friends of mine that I'm training in Pilates, they just laugh! They think it's ridiculous; they have only heard about Pilates when their wives do it after pregnancy to regain urinary control. One friend of mine jokingly asks again and again, "Are you going to pee-pee control hour?" They have no idea that a tough, strong, intelligent German boxer and inventor named Joe Pilates developed the work for men. Joe Pilates took care of his body, and he was as tough as nails! But men don't understand because the advertising of Pilates is primarily about women and femininity. All my friends lift weights and train at the gym. My sister's husband believes he is strong because he can do 50 pushups; while his shoulders may be strong, his legs are relatively weak and his alignment is not centered. Like many men, he has fallen prey to the Western world's ideal, male body image – six-pack abdominals and an overdeveloped chest: it's not about the body as a whole, or health in general. These men don't know that Joe Pilates developed a much better system.

I came to Pilates by default. For five years, I practiced yoga intensively until my teacher retired. Because I've always been active in body conditioning and sports, this was a critical situation. At first, I searched for a new yoga teacher. Then my sister, who had been practicing Pilates for eight years, suggested, "Why not try something else?" A hiker and mountain climber, she took up Pilates to keep up her strength for alpine sports. So I decided to try it. An intensive internet search turned up Amanda Diatta's Pilates studio in Stuttgart, Contrology. I thought, *This looks amazing!*

My first session was in January 2014. With Amanda's expert guidance, I completed a physically and mentally challenging workout unlike anything I had ever done before. Although I was unaware of it at the time, Amanda deftly addressed my misalignment and muscle imbalances with tactile and verbal cues: "Martin's body was relatively strong and flexible when he started Pilates. But he overused his back muscles just to hold various positions. He couldn't activate or articulate his abdominals or move dynamically. His body weight and mass sunk and he was unable to support the movement of his arms and legs." But with each lesson, I continued to improve. Amanda's vivid pictures and images enabled me to identify the correct muscles to facilitate proper movement, muscles that hadn't been trained for a lifetime!

For the last year, I have studied with Amanda three times a week. And what benefits I have reaped! Now I understand that holding in my stomach muscles, activating them, is beneficial. This is new for me. Before Pilates, my stomach just flopped out! When I was first learning, we focused on engaging the abdominals to support the arms and legs. Now this is changing. My abdominals are almost always activated naturally. This is important because they are the foundation and connection between legs, arms, upper back, and chest. This awareness and control make movement more coordinated and responsive with any kind of activity.

Recently I went downhill skiing for the first time since my training began. Skiing *this time* was a very interesting experience because I had much more control. Skiing off-slope is my approach, which means the hill hasn't been prepared by snow plows. I ski toward the mountainside, where snow is deep and challenging to navigate. Pilates training afforded me noticeably more strength, control, and responsiveness. In skiing, it's essential that your mind and body are prepared for quick, coordinated changes. You have to react fast. As a result of Pilates, the time gap between my mental decision and physical response was greatly improved.

In sports, Pilates has clearly enhanced my technical performance and enjoyment. Swimming, which I have done from an early age, is noticeably easier. I have freer movement, improved lung capacity, and increased power. Yet the area wherein I've experienced the most change is in my day-to-day life. I have a sedentary job in a publishing house. Most of the day, I sit at my desk or at a conference table. Since Pilates, I am able to stand from sitting in a chair or get out of my car with ease. My car has seats that are very low to the street. I used to use my hands and arms to push me up. Now, I don't need this anymore.

In addition to physical strength, flexibility, coordination and skill, the right Pilates provides the right positive mental attitude and the right "look." From an aesthetic standpoint, Pilates improves carriage and poise for both men and women. Throughout the course of my profession, I have often been photographed with others in a group. When I see previous pictures of myself, I think, *Oh, my God! My posture was so terrible!* Because I'm relatively tall, 6'2" or 190 cm, I purposely hunched down, leaning forward to have conversations with other people. Amanda helped me understand the benefits of establishing good posture and practicing it. I have come to know that good posture is crucial for health and well-being; it is an extraordinary benefit of Pilates, which you can bring directly from the studio into your daily life. Now I have awareness and control of the Powerhouse to externally rotate my legs, which, in turn, helps lift and carry my torso. This position comes naturally for me, and it feels good. I often think, *Okay, now I can control my posture even if I'm not even thinking about it.* All my muscles are working and under control with little correction.

Nowadays, when I watch other people in a standing position, or walking down the street, or when I notice someone I know in a public setting, I'm surprised how people neglect their own bodies. I'm not suggesting that everyone has to be an athlete. In fact, I'm just an average, healthy person, very normal. I feel sympathy for people who don't practice Pilates because they seem to have little connection to their own bodies. There is a Latin aphorism, "Mens sana in corpore sano," which means "A sound mind in a sound body." Since the word mind is most closely associated with psyche and soul, in my opinion, the body is the soul's home. It's a little philosophical, but perhaps society itself could develop in healthy ways if more people practiced what Joe Pilates called Contrology.

I notice that my colleagues, particularly the men, all have back pain in addition to other kinds of physical difficulties. When men reach 50-55 years of age, they sometimes seem to lose energy and health. At this time in my life, I'm focusing more on these things. Pilates really gives me the sense of having increased energy for tasks of daily living and peak performance. Years before I started Pilates with Amanda, I had an accident from skiing that resulted in shoulder trauma. The injury wouldn't heal, so I always had pain in my shoulder. After three months of Pilates, the pain completely subsided. My body doesn't have any muscle memory of its previous pain. I find this very interesting. Even though I did quite a bit of physiotherapy to reduce pain, it was not successful. The only body conditioning that helped was Pilates.

Pilates gives you a feeling of physical well-being in addition to better body image, which translates into improved self-confidence. There's a sense in which you achieve a more positive mental state. When I couldn't train in Pilates for two weeks, I missed it very much, not solely because of declining posture and conditioning, but because of my state of mind—staying in a good mood. Pilates is for conditioning, skill-building, and day-to-day adaptation for athletics or sports. It is definitely not yoga, which is esoteric, oriented toward spiritual transcendence.

And there's another aspect of Pilates, one that relates to inner ambition for peak performance. Sometimes I think, *Did I really improve this year?* Then I ask Amanda. She replies, "Yes, you did improve," reminding me of the strides I have made, the gradual mastery of more difficult work, and the deeper understanding of the basics. She doesn't give much feedback in this way, though. Her vision of how students can grow and improve and her uncanny ability to motivate and encourage them is enough. I don't think there are many compliments in Traditional Pilates! And that's okay.

Achieving good Pilates technique is challenging. You never have the feeling, *Oh, that's becoming easy now,* but you continue to invest in becoming healthier and more capable. And the training always includes different levels of challenge. Sometimes it's frustrating not to accomplish the right action. During these times, it's important not to lose sight of the overall progress. I recognize that my body has changed in positive ways, yet during the actual lessons, I work hard and try to improve. I am motivated to achieve understanding and technique, so every time Amanda shows me a new exercise I can't do, I try to figure it out. She guides me to find Pilates in my body.

The Work of Joe Pilates begins with a complete system wherein the correct activation of certain muscle groups creates the context to establish proper placement, alignment, and dynamic movement. The body is not conceived as a collection of independent muscle groups, but as a system wherein all muscle groups are working in concert to achieve a particular action or various actions. If you walk into the studio and think, *I want to increase the size of my biceps; I want to flatten my abdominals; I want to improve the shape of my gluteal muscles; I want to lengthen my legs,* exercises and muscles groups become isolated and disconnected from working collaboratively. Although at times we stabilize certain muscle groups and mobilize others, we are not isolating or disconnecting them from the whole body. It's important to remember that all muscle groups are simultaneously working in concert while all concentration is organizing the complete system of mental and physical conditioning. These ideas are central to understanding that one's body is working as a system and not as a collection of isolated functionalities.

The system is brilliant. And it works! Having seen the results in my own body, all I can say is, "I'm sorry for all the people who are not doing Pilates."

About Amanda:

Amanda Diatta's passion for Pilates springs from her love of ballet and swimming—hobbies she has pursued since childhood. Along with continuing education in Spiraldynamik® and becoming a back exercise teacher and certified personal trainer, Amanda completed her Pilates training in 2009 at Pilates New York, in Joseph Pilates' original Method of Body Conditioning. Her teacher, Davorka Kulenovic-Bischoff, was herself a student of Romana Kryzanowska. In 2014, Amanda founded Contrology Pilates Studio in downtown Stuttgart, Germany.

Chapter III

Importance of The Work

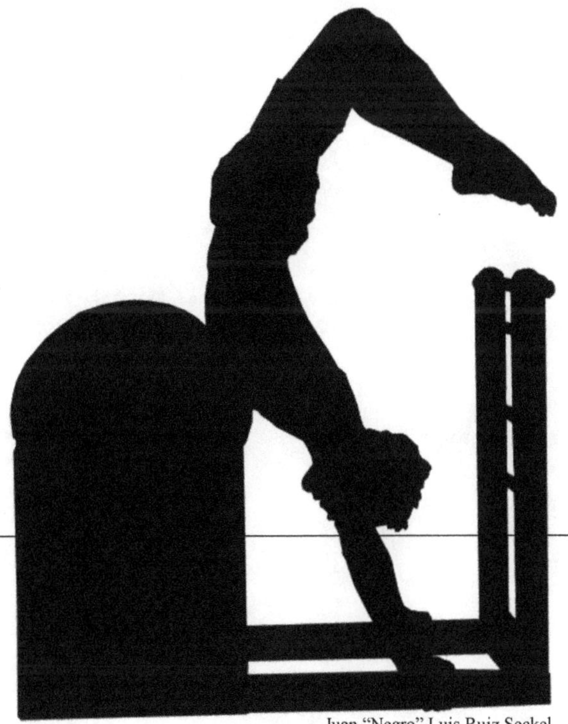

Juan "Negro" Luis Ruiz Seckel

Rediscovering Pilates

By Tony Franco Balongo

No other fitness modality rivals Pilates.

Little did I know when I registered for Dana Santi's Classical Pilates conference several years ago that it would change my life forever! It was my first time working out on Gratz apparatus, and it was my first lesson with Jay Grimes. What a shock when I was suddenly unable to execute exercises I previously thought I had mastered. The realization hit me; my muscular connection to exercises was all wrong. My mental focus was all wrong. My understanding of how and where to begin each movement was all wrong. Although I had learned some theory, in retrospect, it seemed incomplete. And without the right apparatus, it was impossible to do the traditional work or experience the real benefits of Joe Pilates' traditional system. I was hooked! I knew this was what I had to continue doing. So I attended Classical Pilates conferences and studied with classically trained teachers. And I purchased a Gratz Reformer and Wunda Chair, eventually equipping a complete Gratz studio. I am committed to learning the Traditional Pilates technique, the best way to achieve optimal physical conditioning.

My fascination with the authentic work began the moment I saw Kathryn Ross-Nash and Peter Fiasca execute advanced Pilates moves seemingly effortlessly on the Classical Pilates Technique DVDs. Already certified to teach Pilates by Peak, I still knew relatively little about the history of Joe Pilates, the lineage of teachers who trained with the master, and the historically accurate technique. The order of the exercises was similar, yet what I had learned just wasn't the real work. I had to relearn everything. Everything. The process was almost like starting from scratch. Had I started with the classical work, I would have progressed considerably faster. But for the last six years, Jay Grimes, Kathi Ross-Nash, Brooke Siler, Chris Robinson, Dana Santi, Peter Fiasca, Ernesto Reynoso, and Dorothee VandeWalle have guided me on this journey; they have shown me and taught me the historically accurate Pilates Method, which is fierce! Now I am digging into the traditional work at deeper levels and realizing the important benefits derived from it.

When I talk about Classical Pilates, I say, “This is the real work; it’s pure; it hasn’t been changed; it’s how Joe Pilates taught his method and how he wanted it.” The roots of our family run deep, directly back to Joe Pilates himself. It’s how Jay, Kathi, Dana, Brooke, Peter, Ernesto, Dorothee and many other teachers have learned The Work; it’s how these professionals have been teaching me. Like many teachers, I feel strongly about keeping Traditional Pilates intact. I regularly tell my students, “Pilates is becoming more watered down every day; we need more people, more teachers, to keep it alive and keep it true.” Just think about the variety of mutations that exist today—Aqua-Pilates, Aero-Pilates, Yogalates, Physio-Pilates, Basi Pilates, Booty Barre Pilates, Stott Pilates, Piloxing, Polestar Pilates, Fletcher Pilates, Power Pilates, Ball Pilates and many more so-called “styles” euphemistically called contemporary Pilates. The intention is to create commercial trends for financial gain and occupational recognition without learning the depth, breadth, and brilliance of Joe Pilates’ authentic work. Fitness trends come [and go. These derivative styles are for exercise consumers who get easily bored and seek anything new; they are shallow and ridiculous.

The proof is in the pudding! I felt my body change dramatically when I switched to Classical Pilates. Working on the correct apparatus and learning the right exercises provided the vehicle of transformation. In my first lesson with Jay, he didn’t speak to me for about 40 minutes! Not a word. And boy was I nervous. In real time, I learned Jay’s exercise order the way he learned it from Joe Pilates. I just worked my body. He prodded me with his finger here and there, but he never spoke to me until the lesson was nearly over. As I stood there dripping in sweat, Jay remarked, “Look, you’re a strong guy. You’re very athletic. You can do all the exercises. Forget about the fancy stuff, the showy, the flashy stuff. You don’t need those exercises. You’re already strong. You want to make your Pilates better; go back to the basics.” His words haunted me for the next six months, so I focused on fundamentals during every workout.

Before long, I started feeling stronger and more elastic. My body began to look different. My brain felt more connected to my body, providing it with clear directions for moving and correcting. All brain-body wiring was "switched on." As evidence of my improved mind-body connection, under the expert instruction of Kathi Ross-Nash, I was finally able to execute an advanced Pilates Mat workout. Her fierce spirit and indefatigable energy motivated me to dig deep into my Powerhouse and push myself toward the goal of accomplishing Olympic Pilates! I thought to myself, *I want this. I want this.*

It's difficult to perform at this level without someone to guide your body on a regular basis. Living here in Spain, with very few traditionally trained teachers, it may be several months before a qualified teacher instructs my body. So it's possible to pick up bad habits. When this happens, I Skype my lessons. And going back to the basics, as Jay recommended, keeps you on the right path. Sometimes with a particular exercise, I "break it down" like a mechanic stripping an engine. I ask myself, "Is my placement correct? How is the exercise benefiting my entire body? Am I initiating movement from the right muscle groups? If not, how can I work different muscles? What change does this make in my entire body? How is the exercise making me stronger? How is the exercise making me more flexible? Which exercises can help me increase balance and coordination skills for sports?"

On other days, I just get on the Reformer and "go for gold" because I like a vigorous physical workout. When I was 18 years old, I trained with some military personnel. We did interval training—running to the first line, executing as many pushups as humanly possible in a minute. Then we ran to the second line, did squat thrusts and ran back. Next we ran to the third line and did jumping jacks. Another interval was completed at the fourth line, and so on. At the end of the session, whoever got more points won the competition.

There is a very similar dynamic in the classical advanced Pilates Mat workout; no apparatus and no restrictions—like in derivative or contemporary methods—where breathing is micromanaged, where dynamics are nonexistent or uncoordinated, where movement becomes choked to death, and where students can't develop all the positive results of athletic exertion. Most people don't realize that Joe Pilates created his method for normal healthy bodies and athletes. Of course, it's also brilliant for rehabilitation, yet there is a misconception that Pilates is for gentle stretching and elderly people.

This poses a problem when you think of men potentially training in Traditional Pilates. I remember teaching at a studio that had a gymnasium nearby. Men often walked by the Pilates studio, saw the apparatus and practitioners taking lessons, yet they didn't seem to visually "connect" with The Method's intense physically demanding work. I'm sure they thought, *Oh, that's kind of that weirdo stretchy stuff.* I know the perception because many men have essentially spoken these same words.

Because I value my work and want to spread the benefits of Classical Pilates, I had to figure out a way to draw them in. So I decided to offer a free class for men at 12:00 noon on Fridays. These big guys came there thinking, *I'm really strong. I can bench press 160 kilograms; I can squat with 325 kilograms.* Within minutes, I had them dripping in sweat. I brought them to the Wunda Chair, put one spring on, and encouraged them, "Come on, do a pull up." I could almost see blood dripping from their foreheads from the exertion. Then I perched on the pedal, started going up and down, you know, lifting my body up almost like a hydraulic elevator with two legs, then one leg; bop, bop, bop. Their egos deflated, they thought, *What the hell?* Their perception changed. Perhaps they considered, *Maybe I'm not that strong.* Or *I'm strong doing certain things, but this is a totally different situation.* Then I illustrated the uniqueness of Classical Pilates by asking questions to highlight points: "Could you pick up a person with one hand and stand on one leg? You may be able to bench press, but how many times in your life do you utilize that bench press action in your daily life or in skilled physical sports?" My point is that Pilates is directly related to functional fitness; it helps you with anything from fundamental movement to the highest athletic art form—anything. Traditional Pilates will make you strong from the inside out.

When a new client—who has previously trained in Pilates—starts at Valencia Classical Pilates in Spain, they are blown away in good ways! I have heard clients remark, "This has never been so difficult." "I've never sweated so much." Pilates is a kick-ass workout, so a lot of men feel intimidated because they see mostly women doing it. Since they are generally more flexible than men, women often make the exercises look very pretty, and The Method is not as difficult for them. But Pilates need not be pretty, nor should that be the goal of the movement. As long as you're doing the right work, coming from the right muscle groups, "You become Pilates and Pilates becomes you," as Jay Grimes once said.

Besides, practicing Traditional Pilates technique is not a performance; it's a workout. Many people are obsessed with the thought, *How does my Teaser look at the highest point?* They would rather take a picture of their Teaser's final shape instead of gleaning knowledge during the full range-of-motion. There are many pictures on the internet of people demonstrating exercises that are biomechanically incorrect and potentially harmful. I always caution students, "Don't think about making it look pretty. Connect from your core." Every exercise originates from The Center; it's very challenging to gain proper articulation of the abdominals and spine. It doesn't matter what an exercise looks like on another body; yours is unique, so the shape will look different. The most important point is that your body benefits from the traditional work. Sometimes these ideas are difficult for students to comprehend because they see what a particular exercise looks like when another student or teacher executes it. This can be daunting. With every endeavor, though, you have to start from the beginning. If you trust the process, if you trust the traditional system, positive results come. Forcing your way through any given exercise or workout prevents you from achieving proper coordination or quality of movement. You have to find that connection in The Center of your body.

No other fitness modality rivals Pilates, though some may appear similar. The movements in traditional Pilates are fluid and connected: one exercise morphs into another, and another, and another. Think of your entire workout as a single exercise wherein the shapes are constantly changing. You begin in one position then transition into another position within a dynamic system of coordinated movement connections. Transitions are very important in Traditional Pilates technique because they help develop mental conditioning as well as physical coordination. If you achieve all of this perfectly, you might get to a point where you could levitate around the Reformer apparatus!

I teach a wide variety of students who are men: a strong fireman, a triathlete, businessmen, sports enthusiasts, personal trainers, men who are de-conditioned from lack of exercise, as well as men who have herniated discs, knee problems, general muscle tension, and life stress. Their ages range from late teens to 70s. One male client is an author and CEO of a large corporation. An avid huntsman, he has two hip replacements, pronounced kyphosis, cervical fusion, a hiatal hernia, chronic tendinitis and a heart transplant.

Another gentleman, Santos, was the tragic victim of a bomb about 20 years ago; 95% of his body required skin grafts. In addition, several fingers and toes were amputated. During his first session with me, he pulled up his tracksuit pant leg to show me where the fire had destroyed muscle tissue. I felt weak in my own legs, thinking, *Oh, my God. This person has suffered so much, and he wants to try Pilates.* I didn't know where to begin. So I asked, "Is any part of your body experiencing pain symptoms, or do you have any acute symptoms such as inflammation or bleeding?" Since he was pain-free, I suggested, "Let's see what kind of range of motion you have in your body." Clearly, there was life in one foot; there was a little articulation and range of motion, yet he walked somewhat like a penguin. The movement in Santos's body was tense; he slapped his feet when walking. So we began with the basics—how to lengthen his neck, maintaining space between shoulders and neck—how to reduce and distribute tension; and how to articulate each step while coordinating his legs, hips, abdominals, back, and chest. The expression in his eyes on the first day was amazing when I taught him how to move his foot. I'll never forget it. It was a like watching a little kid tasting ice cream for the very first time! Before long, he found a strong connection to Powerhouse muscles; then slowly, but surely, Santos began walking with good posture. His balance improved.

In the beginning, I gave him High Chair exercises: the Press Down, for example, adding the lower-lift heel before bringing the pedal back up. Santos practices that exercise now with arms crossed, not holding the handles. The range of motion in his ankle and his overall movement quality has improved drastically. He walks like Fred Astaire now!

I really enjoy teaching Santos because his case is challenging and complex. And he is one of the most determined people I've ever met; his spirit is resilient and optimistic. Sometimes he asks, "Why didn't I do this before?" I reply, "Well, now you have met me, and we are doing good work; that's how life is sometimes." His wife once commented, "You're never going to give up Pilates." Before studying

The Method, Santos had stopped going for walks with his wife. She enjoyed walking with him, but even a casual stroll caused pain in his shoulders and neck because of tremendous tension.

But you don't see many men getting involved in Pilates, especially young guys. They are obsessed with building bulk and pushing weight. Often when they gain more knowledge and experience in fitness, they become more open to a discipline like Traditional Pilates. Some of the men I teach tell their friends, "Hey, you don't know what this Pilates stuff is. But come to class one day with me, and Tony will kick your ass." The men I teach are sure of themselves; they've got nothing to prove. Yet the marketing and advertising of Pilates is primarily geared toward women, so men avoid Pilates. In addition, the contemporary derivative styles do not provide the strong vigorous workouts that men prefer. And the gyms are doing a lot of damage because they include 25 people in a Mat class; people cannot learn The Method with that many participants, and they are much more likely to get injured.

It's unfortunate that a lot of people still think Pilates is for dancers or that Pilates is only for women and gay men; this stereotype is definitely inaccurate. We're in the year 2014 and this mentality is surprising. Not many people know that Jorge Lorenzo, the 2013 world champion MotoGP driver, does Pilates. And Carles Puyol, the world famous Barcelona soccer team defender, does Pilates. He was physically the strongest man in the Barcelona squad and the strongest man in the Spanish National Football squad. He is a brute! There are many strong guys who do Pilates, and they don't really give a damn what other people think.

Because the traditional system of Pilates is such a powerful technique of strengthening, stretching, and control, it inspires a great deal of passion about developing health and vitality! Ever since I started learning Classical Pilates, I wanted to give people a "jolt of reality" because what's being sold as Pilates is not the body conditioning system that Joe Pilates created. I wanted to help educate the public, to open that window of awareness about Traditional Pilates technique. There are fitness associations in Spain—and throughout Europe—that create macro conventions where hundreds of participants practice the Bosu ball on Joe Pilates' Universal Reformer and the Cadillac. They practice all these biomechanically dangerous exercises, claiming they are doing Pilates, but it's definitely not Pilates. When fitness professionals are ignorant of Joe's traditional system of vigorous exercise, yet they advertise their business as such, it makes me cringe.

I want to share the traditional work the way Joe Pilates created it. My work, though, is just a drop in the ocean. It's very rewarding to organize the Valencia Classical Pilates conferences so people have a positive educational experience with the real work. This way, participants see and feel it. I have a strong sense of urgency to help preserve Classical Pilates, so I created these events; it's hard work, but totally worth it. The energy created during the first year in 2013 was amazing; everyone was on a high. That's because of Peter, Brooke, and Kathi. In 2014 we had three more top-notch classical teachers: Dana, Ilaria, and Ernesto.

Many more people in Spain and Europe need to be exposed to Traditional Pilates, but there are not enough teachers here. Not everybody can afford to fly to the U.S., let alone cover the cost of accommodations. Then there's the expense of taking lessons and classes. So, I want to make Classical Pilates available here in Valencia at a reasonable price. There are a lot of people coming here from other countries. Their eyes, hearts, minds, and bodies have been opened to The Work. I have not forgotten the financial hardship I incurred traveling to the States to study, yet the experience enriched me and enlightened me beyond words. Learning and teaching Classical Pilates technique is a slow process; but it's rewarding, exciting, and transforming. Like anything you want to do well, you have to take your time and be constant. Never stop. If you stop, it's like water when it stops flowing; it stagnates. Classical Pilates will never languish if we continue to study and teach with integrity.

About Tony:

Tony Franco Balongo, London born with Spanish descent, has a background in contact sports, martial arts, and British boxing. It was through boxing that he discovered Pilates while living in Essaouira, Morocco. On returning to Spain, he began taking classes and shortly after then began a training course. The big change came when attending a Pilates conference where he met Peter Fiasca, Kathryn Ross-Nash, and Brett Howard in person.

Affairs of the Heart: Pilates and Cardiac Surgery

By Dr. Roberto von Sohsten & Suzanne Diffine

Opening the chest is integral to restoring health...

Under the best of circumstances, performing cardiac procedures can be tough on a surgeon's back. But interventional procedures compound this strain, as they often require the use of a lead apron to minimize damage from radiation. This 15 pound apron can place pressures of up to 300 pounds per square inch on intravertebral disks. I know this first hand! In 1999, while practicing medicine in Brazil, I regularly performed cardiac catheterizations. During surgery, I could feel the weight of the apron pulling my upper body forward and my lower body down. It wasn't long before my demanding surgical schedule, combined with a lack of physical activity, took its toll on my body. Constant low back pain quickly gave way to an acute, lumbar pain crisis.

Although it took a while, the episode eventually passed. Fearful of a recurrence, I decided to finally heed my wife's advice. For several years, she had been taking Pilates to manage back pain due to scoliosis. At the time, she practiced Polestar Pilates, which significantly reduced the discomfort from her curvature. I thought, *Maybe she is on to something!*

Let's just say I was not the star pupil when I began. Lacking flexibility, upper body strength, and patience, I presented the instructor with a real challenge. Classes were out of the question, so I started with private lessons, focusing on lengthening my spine and strengthening my core. These sessions were unlike anything I had ever experienced before. The workout required more focus and attention to detail, addressing the specific needs of my body. The typical gym workout always seemed to be the same: today let's do all the exercises for the chest or the back or the legs. Pilates, on the other hand, customized exercises and apparatus. Instead of squeezing and contracting, I created space, opened up, released. The emphasis on alignment, lifting, and lengthening soon translated to a heightened awareness of my posture. All day long I corrected myself: stand taller, pull the belly in and up, don't round the shoulders forward. I no longer sat in a chair, perching instead on a large exercise ball to encourage core activation. And I paid careful attention to ergonomics, adjusting the height of my computer and repositioning my head when reading x-rays in order to avoid hyperextending the cervical spine. When using the mouse, I elongated my wrist to prevent carpal tunnel syndrome.

Granted, I was often frustrated when I could not execute certain moves, but generally they were the exercises I needed the most. And the perceptive instructor always ended the session with something I could do well, so I left feeling successful. Most importantly, my back steadily improved. It was clear that Pilates had to be an integral part of my life. The biggest challenge was finding the time to train. Luckily for me, we soon relocated to south Florida, where my wife, Juliana, completed the Romana's Pilates certification. After setting up a small, private studio in our home, she began training me. This was not an easy task, though.

Fortunately, Juliana has a degree in human resources, so she understands the psychology of dealing with the opposite sex. Men generally have a tough time with coordination. And we struggle with any exercise comprised of four or five actions. In general, men need simple directions, one step at time. Since we are less meticulous than women, it is important not to be too methodical, not to break down the exercise too much or you will lose us. I get it now, but in the beginning I just wanted to move. The minute corrections were frustrating. So Juliana just slowed me down, modifying the tempo to give me some happiness. Men must be corrected differently. Don't try to fix every movement or every cycle. Let us do it wrong a few times; then remind us to put pressure on the big toe or stretch the left waist long. If you practice OCD Pilates with men, you will fail. We see it more as a workout and less as education.

In truth, most men are intimidated when they walk into a Pilates studio. Many teachers, studio owners, and directors are women, so we are intruders. Thus, attention to ambience and décor is important in order to make men feel more welcome, more comfortable. Neutral colors, rather than pink, signify that this is not just women's domain. We feel awkward enough, particularly in a class, as The Work is foreign. One-on-one sessions are preferable for a first-timer, as they are so focused that the participant's attention is only on himself.

That said, no matter what the setting or class set-up, I highly recommend Pilates, particularly for post-operative patients. Cardiac surgery can be a daunting proposition. Even the most intrepid souls may feel vulnerable or fragile after bypass or valve surgery. Initially, pain and fear can inhibit movement. For six weeks post-op, patients cannot reach their arms overhead or out to the side. Some are even afraid to brush their teeth or comb their hair. And the families often baby them, compounding the situation. But it is important for patients to get moving as soon as possible, resuming exercise the day after their procedure. Of course, this doesn't mean a patient should go out and run a marathon. For the first few days, just walking around the room or down the hospital corridor is sufficient.

Four to six weeks after bypass, patients can begin cardiac rehabilitation, a structured exercise plan. Exercising 3 times a week with a low workload titrated to age and condition, they slowly progress over 3 months. Although the focus is on cardiovascular exercise, the upper and lower body are worked as well. The target heart rate gradually increases up to 60%-70% age-predicted heart rate and some light weight exercises are incorporated.

Many patients are still fearful at this stage, afraid to exert themselves or increase range of motion. They find reassurance in the fact that professionals carefully monitor them for atrial fibrillation during this first month post-op. However, the medical community is sometimes remiss, focusing on cardiac rehabilitation at the expense of posture or the architecture of the spine. Structural issues caused by the surgery cannot be overlooked. Cardiac procedures change the body forever. As the surgeon dissects the internal, anterior mammary artery for bypass, he lifts the left side of the chest cavity. Significant trauma to this area can often result in thoracic outlet-like syndrome, parasthesia, numbness, tingling, and left shoulder elevation. And respiratory changes occur due to the incision and post-surgical pain. Patients typically do not take deep breaths, thus the respiratory/pulmonary capacity is reduced. All of these issues must be addressed during recuperation.

Opening the chest is integral to restoring health. Some patients are instructed to adopt a protected stance postsurgery to protect the sternum and scar, so as not to disturb the sternal wires. However, the sternum heals very quickly, and the sternal wires are quite strong, binding ribs together. Patients naturally assume a protective stance for the first few days after surgery, as it is quite painful to cough, sneeze, or take deep breaths. Hugging a pillow to splint the chest can alleviate the discomfort. Therefore, initially the habit of hugging a pillow or assuming a caved in attitude of the chest should be discouraged:

- If it doesn't help anymore.
- There really is no more pain.
- The habit can carry forward and patients wind up with some restriction in movement of the chest and shoulders, as well as respiratory compromise due to bad posture.

Instead, after the pain subsides, patients should engage in exercises to open the chest. Because of the way the surgery is done and the exposure of the heart, it tends to be more painful in the left shoulder and scapular area, so most limitation or reduced range of motion occurs in the left shoulder. If the chest is not stretched, creating space, the patient will end up with something akin to thoracic outlet syndrome from a shrinking or overactive trapezius.

The breast stroke is effective in opening the chest. I tell my patients that once the sternum is healed, typically four weeks for the skin incision, then they should walk in the pool and move their arms in a breast stroke fashion to mobilize and stretch the sternum, breaking up adhesions and scar tissue. They wind up with better posture and mobility of the shoulders and upper chest.

After six weeks, there is very little that will disrupt the sternum, so it is time to focus on getting the head and shoulders back, exercising the arms, reaching overhead and mobilizing the scapulae. All too often, therapists avoid larger range-of-motion exercises, preferring low biceps curls, upper body ergometer, or elliptical type upper body movements. Here is where Pilates can step in: using pillows under the head during Reformer or Mat work enable the neck muscles and shoulders to release. Exercises like Rowing and Chest Expansion without springs or Breathing on the Spine Corrector strengthen the upper back muscles and increase range of motion.

The attention to breath during a Pilates workout and the use of the Breath-O-Cizer help increase respiratory/pulmonary capacity and free the body to move more efficiently. Pre-Pilates abdominal work strengthens the core, so patients don't feel so heavy on their feet, so weighted on the ground. Although breathing exercises are an important component of cardiac rehabilitation, isometric exercises may be included as part of a comprehensive exercise program. In general, holding one's breath is not good, as the sudden surge in blood pressure increases peripheral, vascular resistance. It can increase sheer pressure in blood vessels and shouldn't be sustained for a long time. While it is true that this is not advised for someone with cardiac disease, once the patient undergoes bypass or valve surgery, the problem is fixed. The presurgery, physiological limitations no longer exist.

As posture, strength, and range of motion improve, patients can be challenged. Theoretically, four months after surgery, a patient is clear to do any exercise within reason and individual limitation. This includes a minimum of 20-30 minutes of aerobic exercise 5 times a week, light weight training, breathing exercises, opening the chest, and mobilizing and stretching the left shoulder and scapular girdle. There really is no exercise that is contraindicated (unless there was a prior orthopedic or medical condition that precluded a specific movement), as long as the patient had a successful operation and has expert guidance from a trainer who knows how to prevent injury. Obviously, if you were not an athlete before surgery, don't try to be one after, at least not right away! Some postcardiac surgery patients can achieve remarkable gains in overall fitness, however. Recently, I had a very motivated patient, a middle aged woman who had a valve replacement and was able to climb Mount Rainier a few months later! With the proper guidance and education, postcardiac surgery patients can resume an active life, restored to good health by a skilled surgeon and a knowledgeable fitness professional.

About Roberto:

Roberto von Sohsten, MD is a Board Certified Cardiologist. He has offices in the following Florida cities: Atlantus, Wellington and Boynton. His areas of medical interest include hypertension, cardiac prevention, heart failure, coronary and valvular disease, and cardiac imaging. His personal interests include tennis and Pilates.

About Suzanne:

Studio owner of Pilates Rx in Boca Raton, Suzanne Diffine, holds a B.A. and an M.A. in English from the State University of New York at Buffalo. Understanding the connection between a healthy mind and a healthy body, Suzanne has always engaged in some form of physical exercise. A fitness instructor for 30 years, she was also a national Pilates master trainer for Bally Total Fitness and Sports Clubs of Canada.

Carry On!

By Pedro Pereira de Ferreira

> ***...the same exercises are experienced differently by each client.***

It seems like a long time since I began studying Pilates in 1998. At that time, I was attending university in London. One afternoon, I was rushed to the hospital for an emergency appendectomy. My physician recommended Pilates for rehabilitation, as did the physiotherapist, referring me to a studio near the university. Truthfully, I wasn't hooked straight away. Pilates seemed strange, unlike anything I had ever done before. Looking back, I understand that my instructor practiced a derivative interpretation or contemporary form of Joe Pilates' traditional system. Because I did not connect with The Work, I wasn't motivated, but the healthcare professionals insisted I make the commitment. So I began researching the origins of Pilates, the professionals who teach the traditional work, and the man himself—Joe Pilates.

At one point during my research, my teacher, Michael King, recommended a collection of DVDs called Classical Pilates Technique by Peter Fiasca. Once I got my hands on these videos, my path unfolded before me. I took Pilates workshops and completed certifications from several contemporary Pilates programs here in Europe. Each and every certification program referenced Peter Fiasca and his DVDs in their bibliographies. You don't have to be a rocket scientist to recognize the message.

It was time to experience the real work firsthand. My opportunity to meet Peter arose when he taught a workshop in Barcelona. Accompanying him was this feisty woman, Kathi Ross-Nash, who could outperform any man. With these two masterful teachers close at hand, I had a chance to determine whether I was on the right track in my teaching of the classical work. Although I had been teaching for a few years, I was not classically trained, so I had to figure things out on my own. It was gratifying when Peter affirmed that my two students, Sonia and Isabelle, were practicing and training in the right ways. This was a confirmation of the traditional Pilates system and my own instincts as a teacher.

I continued to further my education, traveling to Kathi's American Body Tech studio in New Jersey. Adhering to her punishing schedule, we woke up every morning at 6:30 to complete the advanced Reformer or Mat, continuing workouts during the day; it was killing me! But one afternoon in particular I will remember forever. As I performed the advanced Reformer series, a fellow named Peter walked in. He looked at me for few moments as I struggled with Backstroke. Clearly, I did not "get it!" Then he asked a couple of simple questions which led to a fundamental shift in my approach, "Listen, Pedro, why don't you smile? Enjoy yourself. Let it happen." It worked! Suddenly, I accomplished the Backstroke with the right intention and execution. The entire workout was better.

Until I found industry professionals who were extensively trained in the traditional system, Pilates didn't make sense to me. I couldn't apply the derivative techniques by Peak, Stott, Power Pilates, and The Pilates Institute or other contemporary systems to my life. There was something missing. When I started training in the original work, it was hard. I have strength, agility, stamina, endurance, and I have played many sports. But the derivative techniques put me on the wrong path. I was never able to experience enough confidence to truly trust Pilates. The authentic method enabled me to relate Pilates to the world: the fitness world, the sports world and, of course, the "world" of conditioning my body. Now, even when I'm traveling, it's possible to maintain my health and well-being at peak levels. This is what I know and teach.

The traditional work has inherent wisdom; it develops a level of intelligence wherein you can achieve complete control of your mind and body. Non-Traditional Pilates schools cannot do this because they don't know the real work. Joe Pilates studied the human body and mind in very precise ways. He was a thinker, an inventor, a student, and master of biomechanics. In fact, he studied throughout his career while creating a great system of education in physical and mental conditioning. The Work has changed my life for the better forever. I'm very thankful.

Those who know the authentic work feel the same way. Chris Robinson, a gifted teacher, personal trainer, and martial arts expert, attests to the intelligence of Traditional Pilates; it improves any kind of movement, any fitness technique or sport. For me, it was

CrossFit conditioning and lifting weights in the gym. For Chris, it's been Muay Thai martial arts. As a CrossFit instructor, I never sustained an injury and my stamina remained high because of Pilates. You see, many people who practice CrossFit get injured. I was often asked how I endured conditioning for long periods of time. "It's Pilates," I told them. But Pilates is foundational; the system comes first. Then you apply The Method to other physical disciplines. You shouldn't approach Pilates in reverse; in other words, do not try to teach Pilates based on other movement techniques from sports, martial arts, dance, physical therapy, gymnastics, TRX, CrossFit, or anything else.

The real method takes time to become part of you; you can feel the physical effects straightaway, but the mental benefits, especially for men, may take a longer period of time. As your body develops and your mind deepens its knowledge, however, the benefits become more apparent, effective, and transformative. As Jay Grimes says, "Pilates becomes you, and you become Pilates."

Working to achieve mental and physical progress requires a keen and enthusiastic teacher because it's a complex process that involves struggle and slow transformation. We all need guidance to stay on the right path. When practitioners work out on their own for too long, there's the probability of cultivating bad habits, losing knowledge, and not properly progressing. That's why it's important for me to travel and study with Kathi, Peter, or any of the other world-class teachers. This way, I can ask questions, train, and experience invigorating workouts from trusted sources. As a result, my body stays healthy and strong, on the cutting edge of peak performance. This kind of achievement is important for men; we're physically competitive. We want to win.

But the benefits go far beyond enhanced athletic performance. Because of Pilates, I'm more relaxed and mentally focused when driving a car, an activity that serves as a useful metaphor for managing stress in daily life. Previously, I drove with very tense jaw muscles, preoccupied with distracting thoughts. Now I'm a father with a wonderful young daughter named Maria, who is 18 months old; I'm more relaxed and "present" with her than I would have been before studying Pilates. In general, I'm more at ease, more relaxed with my life, because of decreased tension and improved concentration. My mind is sharper, and I can share knowledge more quickly and clearly with clients. Beyond effectively teaching clients, I have more insight regarding human nature in general; this increased awareness translates into an awareness of emotional/psychological trends of others as well as myself. Remember what Joe Pilates clearly indicated that Contrology is a method of physical and mental conditioning.

When I teach Pilates, I keep it simple and direct. In addition, I learn something from every client. It's curious; sometimes clients are unable, or unwilling, to confess the entire truth of their physical abilities and symptoms. So, as a teacher, I journey with the client and learn important information about who that person is, just like when I read a book; it's a process of discovery. The body in front of you reveals the truth in all of its dimensions. Then you find ways to help the client apply Pilates to their lives, which is a fascinating process for the client and teacher. You provide the client with practical everyday examples as well as specific connections with leisure activities or skilled sports. Pilates is a clever system with innumerable benefits.

Each teacher brings their own history, personality, and life experiences to The Work. Before I studied Pilates, I earned a bachelor's degree in graphic design and a master's degree in art and graphic design. In addition, I studied film design, honing my skills at creating cinematic intrigue, as well as visually accurate and emotionally moving artistic impressions. Working in film design, it's important to create scenes that convey elements of an actor's character. Visual scenery itself can depict essential information about the actor's character. On a parallel track, there are similar elements in Authentic Pilates: there is the client, the equipment, and the creative decision-making process of teachers developing lesson plans using the entire Pilates system of exercises and apparatus. Although we teach a standard repertoire of exercises on traditional apparatus, there's a sense in which clients understand the same "scenery" of technical forms and apparatus in different ways. The uniqueness of each person, and the individual body/mind intelligence, becomes more adaptable and responsive within the same studio environment. Why? Because the same exercises are experienced differently by each client, the teacher provides a different insight, and neuromuscular education itself provides a cumulative and transformative effect. Similar to filmmaking, you've got the same scenery, and the client is like a participant-observer seeing his movement through the lens of his unique perspective, history, intelligence, understanding, mood, sports history, and so forth. From my point of view as the teacher, I encourage students to properly initiate movement from their Powerhouse, feel the intrinsic coordination, and create an aesthetic line that goes beyond their normal expectations.

I never take away from The Work. If someone is unable to achieve certain exercises on the Reformer, I teach them on the Cadillac. If it's better to bring students to the Spine Corrector, then I will teach them on this apparatus. From the very beginning, clients should develop an understanding of the entire Traditional Pilates system using all apparatus, including Pilates Mat. Clearly clients see the benefits because they bring their friends and families to the studio, make new friends and enjoy social time together. It's wonderful to see.

During the past three years, I've been teaching Mat Pilates to a surgeon and orthopedic professor at his house. Recently, he bought the Universal Reformer and Cadillac. The results were immediate: an increase in positive energy during his workouts; a gain in strength, stretch, control, improved mind/body connection, and increased mental sharpness in general. This man has been practicing Mat for three years. Now he understands the benefits of having Pilates equipment to achieve optimal results. For most men, it may take more time to comprehend the usefulness of The Work; it didn't kick for me right away. I could see the physical benefits early on, but I couldn't comprehend the mental benefits in the beginning.

When I think of teaching men, it's important to first let them feel The Work. There is a sense in which you cannot actually teach them. You need to let them gradually learn the movement, finding their own way. Allow men space to explore and hone their understanding of The Work. Although I guide them, I let men discover the movement and progressively go with the flow to the point where they say, "Wow, I found it!" This is the way to teach men; it takes time. Since I teach the authentic system, I give everyone the same work while accounting for individual needs, helping students develop a more responsive body and mind.

But there is a crucial question for everyone who cares about The Work of Joe Pilates. How can we preserve his original intentions and technique to protect the public interest and to pass on The Work to subsequent generations of teachers and students? Almost every certification program in Europe manufactures equipment in addition to teaching derivative movement techniques. Money is the bottom line. Until I found the authentic apparatus that Joe Pilates designed, a major component of The Method was missing for me. But I didn't understand the source of my own ignorance until I was exposed to it. Aside from considering aspects of spring resistance, physical dimension, friction coefficient, and the sheer existence of certain pieces of apparatus such as the Arm Chair and Guillotine, it's essential to experience the entire integrated studio of apparatus that Joe Pilates designed. That's why I brought Gratz equipment to Portugal, opening my own studio. This equipment is essential to preserve The Work. Now Pilates lovers who travel to Portugal can visit Wabi Sabi Studio to train on authentic apparatus.

But it is important to reach a larger audience, to raise awareness of the authentic work. To this end, I created a very successful three-day Classical Pilates conference with Kathi Ross-Nash, Dorothee Vande-Walle and Peter Fiasca; it was the first in Portugal, bringing together students and teachers worldwide. This event inspired so many people. And it was rewarding to share, teach, and continue to learn The Work.

My Studio is the largest, most fully equipped and completely authentic studio in Portugal. Although it might sound odd for an American to hear, I never advertise. The brilliance of Traditional Pilates is this: the bodies of clients naturally advertise their health, strength, vitality, and good posture. Maintaining a truly Authentic Pilates studio is difficult for studio owners who aren't trained well enough to understand the complexity of Authentic Pilates; as a result, they get bored and want to mix other techniques into the schedule. They increase studio income by adding yoga, stretch, barre classes, or other techniques unrelated to Traditional Pilates. Staying true to the roots of The Work, Wabi Sabi draws not only loyal clients, but apprentices seeking to continue their studies with classically trained teachers and authentic equipment. They recognize the breadth of education available to them here. I have studied extensively with Kathi and Peter, who trained with Jay Grimes and Kathy Grant, in addition to Romana. So, I share information that I continue to learn.

Kathi and Peter, as well as other traditional teachers, have encouraged me to continue learning, growing, and enjoying The Work. This is very important to stay connected and on the right path. Otherwise you tend to forget The Work. They were taught by a few teachers who exemplified greatness, yet who are no longer with us – Romana Kryzanowska and Kathy Grant. Their knowledge is invaluable, so I continue to study with them, having recently completed Kathi's program of advanced training. I hope someday to learn from Jay Grimes, as well. These gifted teachers preserve and share the traditional work through their teaching, books, DVDs and inspiring stories, enabling others to learn and live the technique and spirit of Joe Pilates' system of Contrology. I never imagined that my own life would change so much for the better and that Pilates would improve everything else I do. I never imagined that I would help preserve and teach Authentic Pilates to so many wonderful people so they could improve their lives.

About Pedro:

Pedro Pereira de Ferreira is the owner and director of Authentic Classical Pilates® studio in Porto, Portugal. He is Portuguese and was born in Porto, which is a strikingly beautiful northern city where Douro River meets the Atlantic sea and where Port wine is made.

CREDENTIALS

University academic degree in Art & Design.
Certified shiatsu therapist, fitness personal trainer, and CrossFit coach.
Comprehensive certification in Authentic Pilates.
A founding board of director of the Authentic Pilates Union (APU).
Organizer and producer of the first Authentic Pilates Conference in Portugal (2012).
Continued education with professional instructors Kathi Ross-Nash & Peter Fiasca.

TRAINING BACKGROUND

Pedro has been teaching Pilates for more than 15 years. During his academic studies in London, England, he was temporarily injured and recovering from medical surgery, which led him to Pilates. Pedro discovered that Pilates training helped provide physical rehabilitation. He became inspired and decided to complete contemporary certifications, for example, at The Pilates Institute and with Peak Pilates. After discovering the traditional work at True Pilates New York, as well as training with Kathi Ross-Nash, Peter Fiasca and Brett Howard in Barcelona, Spain, Pedro's dedication continued to strengthen and grow. As a result, he focused upon in-depth education and training with Kathi Ross-Nash and successfully completed the Advanced Teacher Training Program. Over the years Pedro has continued to study with several well-respected Classical Pilates teachers as well as teach the traditional system of conditioning at his studio in Porto, Portugal.

Accomplished Man of Excellence

By Miguel Jorge, Jr. & Marian M. Tarín

Perfect Balance of Body and Mind...

The Work of Joseph H. Pilates and the role of Ancient Greece in the history of human culture share a common goal—the creation of the ideal man. Many essential guidelines for living offered in Pilates' writing reflect standards common in Ancient Greece. Pilates' preventive system of physical education, *Contrology*, resembles the Greek concept of *Paideia*, a formula for rearing and educating a man of high ideals. Unfortunately, this invaluable inheritance has been lost, preventing us from enjoying a truly full existence. Therefore, it is beneficial to consider these principles, examining the infinite similarities between these two creations, *Contrology* and *Paideia*.

The Greeks considered education indispensable for the community as well as the individual. Knowledge of self was the pinnacle of human development. Through self-awareness, through the spiritual path, man discovered the objective laws of human nature that foster contemplation and action. The rules that established boundaries for individual behavior as well as society arose from the recognition of these laws. Consciousness of these principles governing the human body and spirit was most important. Thus, Greeks based their education on this knowledge with the purpose of molding men to the ideal of *kalos kagathos*, the "beautiful and good." Similarly, in the Pilates Method, the intuition of the rules that determine structure, balance, and movement of the body provide well-being and self-confidence. The same laws that act upon all things regulate the performances and thoughts of the human being. Joseph Pilates explains:

> Briefly, then, all we need to do in travelling the "road of life" is to trace life itself from birth to youth and middle age to discover that which is responsible for disturbing and upsetting physical and mental equilibrium, that is, balance of body and mind. Then it will be comparatively easy to recognize and understand the causes and to correct them according to

> the infallible laws of nature. In short, study your body, know its good and bad points, eliminate the bad and improve the good and what will be the result? A perfect man physically and mentally![1]

Ancient Greeks put all their efforts into achieving human excellence because it offered the best of all rewards: honor. Aristotle held that true dignity lay not in possessing honor, but in recognizing one's worthiness. In addition to his belief in the value of honor and pride, he considered self-love one of the virtues of a good life. This love of the most perfect individual the spirit can forge constitutes beauty. Aristotle's concept of beauty referred to courageous actions, fair decisions, and brave choices—the general good. For Joe, honor was as important as for the Greeks. He knew that in order to achieve beauty, much more than will is required. Physical and mental efficiency are indispensable:

> Man should bear in mind and ponder over the Greek admonition, "Not too much, not too little." Man's neglect of himself, is destructive of his physical and mental efficiency and tends toward the gradual and progressive weakening of his morale with resulting ever-increasing dishonesty, immorality, loss of all true perspective of his responsibilities to himself and to his fellow man, with corresponding loss of idealism and ethical culture. Those are not mere words—they are facts.[2]

> Perfect balance of body and mind, is that quality in civilized man, which not only gives him superiority over the savage and animal kingdom, but furnishes him with all the physical and mental powers that are indispensable for attaining the goal of Mankind—HEALTH and HAPPINESS.[3]

Greek philosophers are the best source for understanding the concept of balance. In *The Republic I,* Plato examines the balance of body and mind. He espouses a complete education based on music (philosophy, science, or any kind of art) to lessen dependence on the legal system, and on gymnastics to obviate the need for doctors. Exercise is not only important to gain athletic strength; the main goal is to develop the spirit of a soldier. Therefore, the belief that gymnastics exclusively trains the body and music enriches the soul is false. Both educate the soul, but in different ways. Thus, it is important to find the balance between the two, without giving preference to one at the expense of the other. An education focused solely on gymnastics cultivates excessively the hardness in men and an education based exclusively on music makes men too delicate. Plato believed in a paideia, conceived as an inseparable unit, where the education of the body and the spirit were the forces of human nature's wisdom. Pilates affirmed the importance of this principle:

> They (the ancient Greeks) fully understood that the nearer one's physique approached the state of physical perfection, the nearer one's mind approached the state of mental perfection. They knew that the simultaneous and co-equal development of one's ability voluntarily to control one's body and mind was a paramount law of nature and that the unequal (abnormal or subnormal) development of either the body or the mind, or the neglect of either or both, would result in the complete failure to realize the very first law of civilization —(preservation of life)—the attainment and maintenance of one's bodily and mental perfection.[4]

The science of medicine provides us with evidence for a new philosophical conception of human nature and, therefore, for the creation of the most perfect man. Nature imposes rules that must be understood in order to live correctly in a state of perfect health. Plato, as well as Aristotle, believed that in order to be virtuous, man must embrace excellence in body and spirit. And Joseph Pilates shared this opinion. He created his Method based on the observation and understanding of the laws of nature. His corrective system develops the body, mind, and spirit:

> To one who has devoted the major portion of his life to the scientific study of the body and practical application of nature's laws of life as pertaining to the natural development of coordinated physical and mental (normal) health and the prevention, rather than the cure of disease...[5]

The Greek philosophers found a pattern for human conduct in the science of medicine. They employed the medical terms of excess and defect to provide humans with a guide to appropriate moral behavior. Aristotle defined this principle as a "just middle." This is not an exact point between ends, but a middle ground that varies with the individual; one's moral behavior should lie somewhere between too much and too little.

Consequently, the science of medicine offered a valuable contribution to the spiritual development of man: maintaining health. Fundamental to the Greek physicians' doctrine was the belief in the interdependence of all things in nature. They strove to understand the function of a unit within the group. The balance between the parts or forces of the organism constituted, in medical terms, the natural state or normal health. In a healthy state, it was one's own nature that imposed balance or the "just middle." Nature acts in agreement with the law of symmetry. Thus, Plato considered strength, health, and beauty virtues of the body and mercy, bravery, moderation, and justice, the moral virtues of the spirit or soul. The symmetry of these forces was the foundation for achieving perfection in mankind.

Consequently, when illness altered the body's equilibrium, the doctor's task was to find out how to facilitate the natural healing process. Symptoms of disease, such as fever, represent the beginning of the recovery process, evidence that nature helps itself; we have the capacity to heal ourselves, to prevent disease. The objective of medicine is the elimination of that which causes pain and suffering. But, often nature can achieve this by itself.

In order to preserve the normal state, the Greeks emphasized education in medical culture; this knowledge helped the individual to prevent disease or hasten recovery by understanding and following the doctor's instructions. The goal of effective treatment could not be achieved if the individual was not an active participant, conscious of the doctor's purpose. Ancient doctors educated society in hygiene or diet. This was much more than ordering foods; it was a daily regimen, which included guidelines for good habits and mechanisms to deal with external forces impacting the individual.

This related directly to gymnastics. Exercise was important in the lives of Greek men. The gymnast, expert advisor in the care of the body, was the doctor's precursor. When doctors first considered the concept of diet, they worked in tandem with gymnasts. In the fourth century B.C., the famous doctor Diocles of Carystus created a daily medical plan, consisting of morning and afternoon sessions at the gymnasium. In his writings, he omitted any details of the training, leaving this to the gymnast. However, ancient dietetic works, such as *About the Diet*, note that eventually the science of medicine tried to supplant the field of gymnastics, but it didn't take long to establish clear jurisdictions. When needed, the doctor referred to the gymnast for advice because he met regularly with individuals. Such specific and personal information is necessary for medical treatment to be precise and effective, and a doctor cannot obtain this kind of knowledge from infrequent visits.

Ancient Greek works included many guidelines related to exercise, diet and other routines, based fundamentally on symmetry. The physical culture, as Greek gymnasts and doctors conceived it, was something spiritual. They encouraged men to rigorously observe a healthy balance of the physical exertion. This balance created the essence of well-being and physical perfection. However, the concept of health applied to more than just the individual. On a universal level, equilibrium and harmony were the basis that created the "good" and the "fair" in all aspects of life.

In order to achieve this goal, some instruction was necessary. Diocles' work details a daily routine to achieve a worthwhile life. In his regimen, one rises at sunrise. After elimination, oil is massaged on the body to lubricate the joints. This is followed by a walk before or after breakfast. The rest of the morning is spent working or taking care of one's responsibilities, followed by a requisite exercise session. The duration and intensity of the exercise varies with the individual's age. The young go to the gymnasium and adults or the infirm enjoy a public bath or a sunny place, again massaging oil into the body. They never receive a massage, as the vigorous movements required to perform the massage constitute exercise. A light lunch to aid digestion is followed by a short nap in a dark, well-ventilated place. Then, time is reserved for necessary tasks; and after a small break, the gymnastics of the second half of the day are completed. The principal meal follows.

The goal was to instill healthy habits to preserve the normal and natural state of the human race. Therefore, doctors sought to teach these skills to healthy Greek men, the true object of their attention, instead of focusing all their effort taking care of the ill. Joe Pilates shared this opinion: "The man who uses intelligence with respect to his diet, his sleeping habits, and who exercises properly, is beyond any question of doubt taking the very best preventive medicines provided so freely and abundantly by nature."[6]

We should have the utmost respect for medicine, science, and research, which are indispensable to society. By the same token, we must be responsible for our own health. Plato affirmed that the two indicators of a poor paideia were the courts of justice and the health care institutions. He maintained that the growth of these institutions was anything, but the pride of civilization and the goal of education was to render these institutions superfluous. Joe shared this opinion:

> As civilization advances, we should find the need of prisons, lunatic asylums and hospitals growing steadily less and less. But do we find this to be the case in this era? Certainly not! Teach the human race to care properly for itself and you will do away with these abominable institutions.[7]

We should view this statement as constructive criticism, instead of supposing that the intention is to offend lawyers, judges, doctors, nurses, scientists, or any other related professionals whose work is so important. Objective scientific data is essential to establish a universal guide for health. An entity like the World Health Organization performs this function, but there is an important aspect of health that does not fall under its purview. This is precisely where the Pilates Method takes over. Pilates understood that in order to reestablish balance, to be truly healthy, every human being must follow a different path. For this reason, he created a variety of exercises and apparatus, all necessary to address each individual's issues. By gaining self-knowledge, correcting weaknesses, improving strength and flexibility and exposing the body to greater challenges, we can reach our normal state—a state of balance, free of strain or stress, free to move without restrictions. This is achieved through The Method's dual focus, developing a strong center extending into a two-way stretch. This constant energy guides the body through three dynamic directions: flexion and extension, lateral movement, and rotation. When the body is free of tension, then energy is transferred from one place to another, allowing our system to do what it naturally is meant to do. We are designed to heal ourselves, to restore balance, if we listen to our bodies.

Just as Joseph Pilates healed the body, the ancient Greek philosopher Socrates was the medic of the soul. Through his *theory of ideas*, he examined man's moral world, focusing on such concepts as *fairness, goodness and beauty*. Viewing *health* as a reflection of the laws of nature, he believed an analysis of the cosmos must be based on natural human order. During physical training breaks at the gymnasiums, Socrates engaged in dialogues or conversations in the form of questions. According to Plato, Socrates liked to compare his dialogues to getting undressed in front of the doctor or the gymnast to be examined before physical activity. The dialogues offered him the opportunity to observe youth; and, consequently, many citizens sought his advice regarding their children's education. His questions inspired and elevated those around him, and the intensity of the conversations made the gymnasiums a popular place to meet. Here seeds of new thoughts were sewn. The *gymnastics of contemplation* was born, and it did not take long to be considered a new form of paideia.

In his dialogues, Socrates encouraged men to examine their lives, to determine what made one's life worthwhile. Concerned that they sought material gain instead of spiritual enlightenment, he urged them to invest their efforts in search of the good, elevating the soul. Joe agreed:

> The mistreated body, mindful of his past neglect, eventually exacts its repayment in full with interest in the form of leaving business men their fortunes to contemplate, but denying them the benefits and enjoyments that accrue to other men of wealth blessed with normal health.[8]

The development of the spirit and, consequently, all humanity relies on objective knowledge. Beliefs that help us become better individuals may not provide economic benefit, but they are valuable. Rousseau notes that ancient Greek legislators discussed culture and virtue, while our politicians talk about commerce and money. Our educational system is based on capitalism; people are educated to be productive. Greek society pursued the collective goal of happiness. This was achieved through the individual journey of self-knowledge. Joseph Pilates concurred:

> After completing their school day studies, they (children) are compelled to study professions or accept such occupational employment as their parents decide in their "infallible wisdom" is best for them and except in rare cases of rebellion against parental authority, the "victims" resign themselves to their destined fate to the detriment of themselves and society.
>
> Children are impregnated with the thought that success is measured with the acquisition of money and therefore, their aim should be to become rich as quickly as possible.
>
> Millions upon millions live from the cradle to the grave without really knowing themselves and without really knowing what it is all about. If they are familiar with the Greek adage, "know thyself," it is not practically applied to themselves.
>
> These children....slowly sink to a low level, never experiencing the thrills of life, never experiencing the glory of successful accomplishment, and never enjoying the fruits of overflowing vitality and health that should be theirs if taught the problems of life and the proper control of the body.[9]

It is sad to see most human beings chasing after material gain, unaware of their damaged spirits and uninterested in their surroundings. Their constant desire for power precludes an appreciation of the joys of day-to-day existence or the beauty in life. We impoverish ourselves, while believing we are rich. The love of wealth destroys knowledge and morality, essential values for civilization.

Socrates was a staunch defender of this belief. By seeking *truth* and *valor*, man nurtured the soul, the ultimate goal of mankind. But the psyche is not separate from the physique; body and soul must be viewed in concert. The soul is elevated through bravery, consideration, justice, and mercy; the body achieves perfection through health, strength, and beauty. The symmetry of physical and spiritual excellence is *health.* Clearly, Pilates understood this:

> With body, mind, and spirit functioning perfectly as a coordinated whole, what else could reasonably be expected other than an active, alert, disciplined person? Moreover, such a

> body freed of nervous tension and over-fatigue is the ideal shelter provided by nature for housing a well-balanced mind that is always fully capable of successfully meeting all the complex problems of modern life. Personal problems are clearly thought out and calmly met.
>
> The acquirement and enjoyment of physical well-being, mental calm, and spiritual peace are priceless to their possessors if there be any such so fortunate living among us today. However, it is the ideal to strive for, and in our opinion, it is only through Contrology that this unique trinity of a balanced body, mind, and spirit can ever be attained. Self-confidence follows. The ancient Athenians wisely adopted as their own the Roman motto: "Mens sana in corpore sano" (A sane mind in a sound body). And the Greeks as a people displayed even greater wisdom when they practiced what they preached and thus came nearest to achieving its actual accomplishment. Self-confidence, poise, consciousness of possessing the power to accomplish our desires, with renewed lively interest in life are the natural results of the practice of Contrology. Thus we achieve happiness.[10]

Joseph H. Pilates' motivating words should inspire us to seek individual excellence. But it is not an easy endeavor; it requires effort and will. In fact, without proper guidance, success is not guaranteed. That is why we must be responsible for ourselves, find out who we are, and develop the self-confidence that ensures integrity in our behavior. Through Contrology, values are acquired and priorities are reestablished. In ancient times, these standards were appreciated. Respect was measured through dignity; happiness followed self-esteem. If we reincorporate this educational system in our modern society, return to our origins, and reestablish simple rules based on the order of nature, healthy, capable, loyal, tenacious individuals will triumph in the fight for survival. Pilates observed the animal kingdom and understood that, although reasoning distinguishes us from the savage, we cannot abandon our innate nature. We must find the balance between our physical and spiritual capabilities to develop ourselves completely. Then, we can attempt whatever we want.

About Miguel:

An avid athlete, Miguel enjoys judo, soccer, surfing, and water polo. In 1988, he received his master's degree in physical education from the Santa Cecilia dos Banderantes University in Sao Paulo, Brazil. After completing postgraduate work in Sport Training at the same faculty, he became an associate professor of Masculine Rhythmical Gymnastics. Following his stint as a university teacher, he competed in the discipline of Aerobics. In 1991 and 1992, he won the Silver medal in the Brazilian Aerobic Championship. As a coach, in 1996, Miguel's trainees won gold medals in the European Aerobic Championship in Helsinki, Finland. The same year, his team repeated a first place win in the World Aerobic Championship in Orlando, Florida. During this period, Miguel presented at fitness conferences in Brazil, Argentina, Spain, Germany, Italy, France, Hungary, and Korea. In 1993, he received the official Certificate of Reebok as coach of the "Body Walking" program by the USP University. After moving to Spain, he opened a gymnasium in Barcelona, called Studio Olympia. It wasn't long before he began studying Classical Pilates, traveling to Brazil and the U.S. In 2009, he received Pilates Method Alliance certification. From 2004-2010, Miguel was teacher of the Pilates Certification Program at Orthos Barcelona. Always eager to learn more, he travelled to Los Angeles, California, and was certified by elder Jay Grimes at Vintage Pilates. In 2013, Miguel received his certificate of 'The Work'.

During his apprenticeship, he also trained regularly with founders of Vintage Pilates, Sandy Shimoda and Karen Frischmann. Co-owner of the studio PILATISTIC, Old School Pilates (Centre Pilates Tiana), Miguel believes in the importance of learning more every day. He continues to travel and study with the best Traditional Pilates teachers throughout the world. Now he's thrilled to start a new apprenticeship next to another world renowned teacher, Kathryn Ross-Nash and her program Pilates Professional Advanced Teacher Training 2017 The Red Thread®.

About Marian:

Marian began practicing Pilates while she was studying journalism at the International University of Catalonia. She was so amazed at how The Method challenged her body that when she received her master's degree in 2004, she enrolled in teacher training. Studying with some of the best Classical Pilates teachers in Brazil and America, in 2009 she received her certification from the Pilates Method Alliance. Several years later, she opened a studio in Barcelona, co-owning PILATISTIC, Old School Pilates (Centre Pilates Tiana). Due to her fervent interest in improving her professional skills, she undertook a course of study with elder Jay Grimes at Vintage Pilates in Los Angeles, California, receiving her Teacher's Program Certificate in 2013. During her apprenticeship, Marian also trained with the founders of Vintage Pilates, Sandy Shimoda and Karen Frischmann. A year later, Marian received an invitation from Jay Grimes to participate in Teaching The Work 2015-2016, a highly selective program where she continued improving her skills and developing her own style as a teacher. Marian is honored to be one of the few instructors in the world who has completed this exclusive mentorship.

In parallel, she has collaborated in all the editions of the Valencia Classical Pilates Conference, translating the words of some of the guest teachers, such as Peter Fiasca, Lori Coleman-Brown, Chris Robinson, and Dorothee Vandewalle. Presently, Marian is presenting at the Classical Pilates Conference Brazil 2017. Due to her incessant will to delve into the Method, Marian is traveling to New York to mentor under worldwide renowned Kathryn Ross-Nash through her program, Pilates Advanced Teacher Training 2017, The Red Thread®.

REFERENCES

[1] Pilates, Joseph H., Your Health. Presentation Dynamics Inc., 1998-2008, 24. First published by Joseph H. Pilates, 1934.
[2] Pilates, Joseph H., Your Health. Presentation Dynamics Inc., 1998-2008, 23. First published by Joseph H. Pilates, 1934.
[3] Pilates, Joseph H., Your Health. Presentation Dynamics Inc., 1998-2008, 2. First published by Joseph H. Pilates, 1934.
[4] Pilates, Joseph H., Your Health. Presentation Dynamics Inc., 1998-2008, 36. First published by Joseph H. Pilates, 1934.
[5] Pilates, Joseph H., Your Health. Presentation Dynamics Inc., 1998-2008, 6. First published by Joseph H. Pilates, 1934.
[6] Pilates, Joseph H., and William John Miller, Return to Life Through Contrology. Incline Village, NV: Presentation Dynamics, Inc., 1998, 17.
Originally Published by J.J. Augustine, 1945.
[7] Pilates, Joseph H., Your Health. Presentation Dynamics Inc., 1998-2008, 22. First published by Joseph H. Pilates, 1934.
[8] Pilates, Joseph H., Your Health. Presentation Dynamics Inc., 1998-2008, 14. First published by Joseph H. Pilates, 1934.
[9] Pilates, Joseph H., Your Health. Presentation Dynamics Inc., 1998-2008, 26. First published by Joseph H. Pilates, 1934.
[10] Pilates, Joseph H., and William John Miller, Return to Life Through Contrology. Incline Village, NV: Presentation Dynamics, Inc., 1998, 23. Originally Published by J.J. Augustine, 1945.

BIBLIOGRAPHY

Jaeger, Werner. Paideia: los ideales de la cultura griega. Fondo de Cultura Económica, 1962. (Original Title: Paideia, Die Formung des Griechischen Menschen. First published in 1933.)

Ordine, Nuccio. L'utilità dell'inutile. Nuccio Ordine and RCS Libri S.p.A, Bompiani, Milàn, 2013.

My Return to Life

By Rafael Luis Fiorini

...there is no better way to fight weakness than strength.

My life can be summed up in one word: reinvention. It has been a continuous struggle to recreate myself. A conscious effort not to be like my parents. Not to be like my friends. To be myself. Completely.

When I was young, I had no notion of myself. I was just a product of all the fear and humiliation I suffered. Afraid of my parents and siblings. The object of derision at school. Teachers called me "trash," destined to be a nobody. And what horror I endured at the hands of my classmates. Threatened and beaten for being fat and clumsy, I ran home crying most school days, wondering what I did to deserve their ridicule. But deep down inside I knew.

Academically, I struggled. Athletics were a laughing matter. But I was good at playing drums. The rage of punk rock spoke to me. The anger that filled every moment of my life made me wild and unpredictable. I played drums with a strange fury. Other kids thought I was crazy. Actually, I hated myself back then. All I wanted was to make good friends, "fit in," and develop more confidence if someone started a fistfight with me in the hallway between classes.

As the years passed, I learned to keep it all inside. Sometimes I talked to other classmates who had similar challenges. Some of them today are the best people I've ever met. One individual is a chap who frequently made bad decisions that seemed strange. I thought to myself, just treat him with respect, and you will find a loyal friend forever. Even with friends, school sucked.

Somehow I survived, graduating and then enlisting in the military. Fearing a repeat performance of my school experience, I trembled with fear at the first sight of my army advisor, Captain Wagner. He was an imposing figure, a hulk of a man. Terrifying. No one dared talk out of turn in his class. Captain Wagner immediately saw that I was not in good physical shape, and one Friday during October he cornered me, then asked, “Have you ever experienced physical training?” “No,” I replied, quaking in my boots. Without a word, he spun on his heels and walked away. The following Monday after work, Captain Wagner said, “I am going to teach you how to train.” As part of his training program, he would surprise-punch my abdominal muscles when I walked down the school hallway. Once I could withstand the beatings, we had an understanding.

Wagner showed me some basic exercises. I watched as if I had never paid attention in my life. I didn’t want to ruin that chance. As the weeks passed, Captain Wagner lived up to his promise, thrusting his fist in my stomach from time to time as he passed me in the hallway. The other soldiers didn’t know what to think. Weeks passed and my performance improved. I could feel the force growing inside my body. Just before Christmas recess, I was on my way to class, and suddenly Captian Wagner appeared, striking me squarely in the chest. I laughed and kept walking. “Now you can look at yourself in the mirror,” he announced walking away. I rushed home, ran to the bathroom and slowly lifted my shirt. There in the mirror I saw a body, not just the shell that held my stomach and my heart. Bulging biceps. Chiseled chest. I felt strong. It was the first time I remember having a sense of myself. I had finally achieved something. And no one could ever take that away from me...or so I thought.

When I left the army, I enrolled in university. But my mind wasn’t focused on studying. What I really liked was to hit the road playing drums in rock and roll bands. I lived with wild abandon. Sure, I had a life full of troubles, but I enjoyed every part of it. I enjoyed it too much. Lessons learned in the army faded into my past.

I had a serious addiction, and it took time for me to accept. This admission was the first step in recovery. I had to accept it. And ask for help. I was afraid of being criticized and seen in a negative light. Yet, it was therapeutic to admit shortcomings and have the courage and conscience to improve. I started living healthier and making better choices. Life can be complicated. There are some temptations that can be seductive, yet illusory, like a mirage in the desert. I have learned that love and happiness come from within, and they are essential to freely share and blessedly receive. Before it was my way to fight emotional pain. Troubling times can be part of life for everyone, to some degree, yet they can also be a transformative force.

The answer to my problems came in the most unexpected place. Despite many challenges, I completed my degree in physiotherapy. One day I attended a lecture/demonstration about Pilates. My interest piqued, I obtained a copy of "Return to Life Through Contrology," and I devoured it. As I read the words of Joseph Pilates, my path unfolded before me. Not long after this fateful moment, academic degree in hand, I began searching for Classical Pilates in Brazil.

After my first class, I knew I had found the perfect antidepressant. No side effects. Only the body and the mind uniting to awaken to their true potential. Now it was impossible to go back. It took me 27 years to discover Classical Pilates, but I finally experienced a real return to life.

As I continued to train and study, I learned of Peter Fiasca. Reading his books and watching his videos only deepened my understanding of the work. His words and movements were so clear; I understood exactly what he was trying to teach me. It was like seeing with his eyes and his heart. What an inspiration! When I finally had the honor of meeting him, he became my mentor, friend, and teacher. Peter encouraged me to dive deeper into the Pilates system at Metropolitan Pilates, the world-class education center licensed by the State of Washington. There I studied extensively with Master Teacher Dorothee VandeWalle, whose iron hands and eagle eyes overlook no detail, no matter how small.

Teachers like Peter and Dorothee inspire us to develop ourselves. They make us recognize our strengths and focus on our weaknesses in order to grow both mentally and physically, for there is no better way to fight weakness than strength. And they encourage self-awareness, a conscious examination of one's actions and thoughts, for nothing good is achieved without work and dedication.

I carry these lessons with me in my own teaching. Many men come into the studio for different reasons, with different goals in mind. While I sought to overcome pain and loneliness, others look to improve their balance, flexibility, coordination, posture and core strength, reduce stress, or resolve low back pain and muscle imbalances. No matter what the reason, the traditional system of Pilates provides added benefits; it sharpens the focus in men, enhances the ability to concentrate, and develops inner strength and confidence. The body must bend to the will of the mind. Anyone who doubts this fact need only attempt training while on "automatic pilot." Impossible!

Once an individual understands Pilates technique, he or she will experience a more integrated sense of self. It is not a bad idea to sometimes challenge your client with advanced exercises, even if they are not executed with complete accuracy. Men want to move without too much correction. Movement reinforces muscle memory over the long term. And we cannot progress unless we practice new challenges. Men certainly appreciate being challenged!

Experiencing resilience in mind and body are important; and it's essential to rely upon our strengths on a daily basis. In a real sense, people are frequently "separated" from their own bodies. We are often temporarily whole or integrated. Our bodies are weakened by stress. Our minds are assaulted. In the midst of living complex lives in a complex modern world, devoting time to Pilates training can help clarify everyday stress in everyday living. Traditional Pilates technique always sets you straight and tells the truth.

It has taken years for me to fully appreciate the value of lessons I learned in Classical Pilates. In this journey, I will continue to deepen the knowledge as I study, train, and teach. When the body is strong, the mind is keen and perceptive. Yet Pilates has given me more than physical strength and mental conditioning. The traditional system of Joe Pilates has taught me to live.

About Rafael:

Rafael Luis Fiorini is an accomplished physiotherapist and the owner-director of Pilates Estúdio Controle E Arte in Peruibe, Brazil. He achieved comprehensive certification under the directorship of Dorothee VandeWalle at Metropolitan Pilates in Seattle, Washington, U.S. Throughout the years, Rafael also trained with Junghee Won, Peter Fiasca as well as Kathryn Ross-Nash.

Chapter IV

Finding the Way

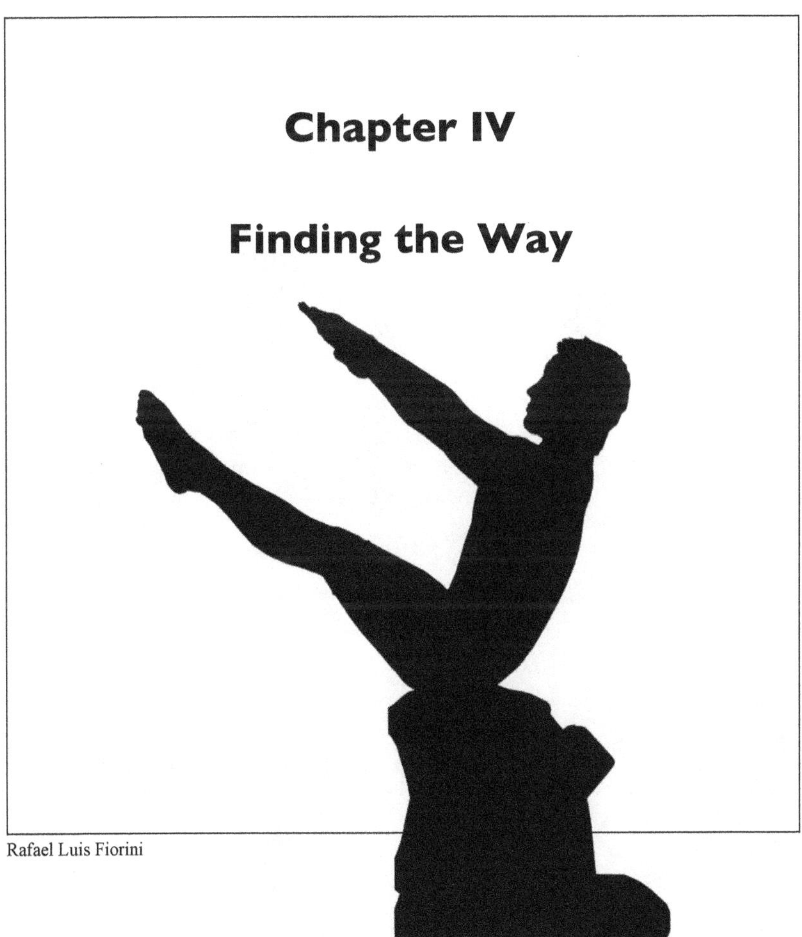

Rafael Luis Fiorini

Working from the Inside Out

By Juan "Negro" Luis Ruiz Seckel

> ***...be mentally disciplined and in charge of your own body.***

At first glance, Pilates seems to have nothing in common with acting. But I discovered firsthand the myriad ways in which The Method benefits professional actors like me. It's imperative that actors learn, grow, increase their awareness, and sharpen their skills daily. One important part of acting is having knowledge of the body. To that end, I embarked on a search for an exercise modality to improve my mind/body connection. Since my brother is a Pilates trainer, I had heard of this system of body conditioning. But from the advertising and pictures I observed, I envisioned Pilates as some kind of dance or movement class. When my brother offered to introduce me to the system by giving me a lesson, I agreed. That night, after finishing the session, I slept soundly for the first time in many years. Previously, I sometimes required prescription medication in order to get a good night's sleep.

As I continued my training, I noticed a significant improvement in my concentration; this was quite surprising, as professional actors always possess exceptional mental focus. And it turns out that practicing concentration in every lesson is what helped me sleep better. By mentally focusing on developing better alignment, strength, and flexibility, I was able to relax and be more fully "present." So I became passionate about traditional Pilates. I wanted to gain more knowledge and achieve more technical skill in the system. The more frequently I trained, the better my concentration and sleep became. These benefits translated into improving simple activities like walking. This increased awareness also improved my ability to make positive decisions.

I have a lot of energy, which at times can be intense. And I'm focused. With every endeavor or activity, I give it my all, investing my full attention and energy, "throwing it to the basket" every day. So I need time for the discipline of Pilates to help guide and structure my energy and keep me centered. The Work definitely enhances my acting technique; I am better able to interpret scripts or move correctly in order to portray a particular character. It also helps me with improvisation. Pilates' intelligent physical conditioning prepares me to accomplish anything. In daily life, we communicate a lot of information through the body. We "speak" through the body, conveying our feelings and the composition of our character. Sometimes in acting, you don't even need written text. You communicate your experience, emotions, and ideas through nonverbal movement.

One day my acting teacher announced, "You will be tree number four." Confused, I pondered the purpose of this exercise. "You don't have written or spoken text," he continued; "You don't have anything except your body. You're tree number four; that's it." Uncertain of his intention, I began to doubt myself. Then I realized, if I'm a tree, there is reason, a purpose. In this particular role, the tree moves through the entire play without verbal or nonverbal communication. Here is where Pilates conditioning was essential. My muscles were strong, supple, lengthened. The Pilates work helped me become the swaying tree. Once I understood the purpose of the exercise, I started to see that written or spoken words were not necessary. Sometimes you don't have to say anything; just be in control of yourself. My new-found confidence and enhanced technique took my acting to a new level. I could potentially become anything or anybody in a role or in life. It just takes focus, feeling the unity of body, mind, and spirit, as Joe said. For the first time, they were no longer separate entities.

I enjoy walking and riding a bicycle. I have a powerful Moto Guzzi for transportation and fun. But I always have my Powerhouse muscles activated and on alert. I feel them working all the time: when I wake up in the morning, when I do a big stretch, when I take a big breath. Just like that song, "I've Got the Power." My body has balance, stamina, control, strength, alignment, energy, readiness for action; it's amazing to feel these qualities and use them for action…or inaction! When it's time for sleep, I can say to my body, "Hey, we need rest." And it responds.

Classical Pilates is an excellent foundation for mental and physical well-being, challenging you every day. It is not a system in which you can learn everything; in fact, it's downright impossible to completely master all the athletic challenges. But you learn as much as possible, earning your weapons of strength, flexibility, and art of control; then you go out and play. It's like being prepared for battle, the battle of daily living. You have important tools and powerful weapons that keep you alive, so you can go into the world. It's survival; it's life. Sometimes you're crossing a street when a car approaches too closely, yet the muscles of a mountain lion are in charge of your body. You're ready for action. The traditional work is about physical and mental resiliency and self-knowledge.

In a sense, Pilates saved my life. During college, I attended five institutions of higher learning. At each one, I felt I didn't have the space or understanding to tap my creativity or motivation in the way that society demands. Frustrated, I searched for ways to harness my energy, to let my body do what it felt. If only I had known about Pilates then. What a different experience college would have been!

But The Work has changed in recent years. Joe Pilates was a man —an inventor, boxer, and circus performer. His original studio was a real gym with the scent of sweat in the air. People worked out... hard. Today, instructors often focus too much on creating ideal forms through placement and alignment at the expense of vigorous athleticism. It's common knowledge among traditional teachers that Pilates' system of conditioning has become too careful, too slow, too feminine. Think of the advertisements and marketing ads depicting women in elegant body position, extending their legs in ways that 99% of men cannot achieve. They're smiling. They're relaxed. They're pretty and not really working. As soon as men see photos like that, they believe that Pilates is a women's workout or some effortless, feminine stretching technique. So men aren't interested in Pilates.

In contrast to the typical Pilates clientele, most of my clients are men because I actively recruit men. As a man, I demonstrate the intense Traditional Pilates system and its physical discipline. Men can see that I am working hard. Most men work out in a different way from women; they talk less and physically push their bodies more. Men come into the studio and say, "Okay, let's go; we have one hour." They are more basic in that way, more direct. As a teacher, it's natural for me to take control of the lesson, guide men with strength, and be direct with instructions. They understand and just work. Sometimes I find it's more challenging to teach women, although there are many women who work with strong athleticism just like any man. For the most part, when I'm teaching, I tend to be stricter with women because they periodically disconnect from the hard physical work and begin to talk about various pleasantries. With men, I am more powerful.

In a real sense, the Pilates profession would improve if more men became teachers. Unfortunately, most men don't understand the phenomenal mental and physical benefits. So, it's part of our work to encourage them to try Traditional Pilates. The Method gives men many qualities and skills they don't learn at the gym; it's one thing to have muscles, to increase muscle mass, to build stamina. But it's quite another task in Pilates to control your muscles to accomplish dynamic complex movement with few repetitions and simultaneously increase responsiveness of the central nervous system and brain. After learning the system and getting a good workout, many clients comment, "Man, what happened to me? I feel my whole body." That's The Method. I don't do anything special. I just teach the Traditional Pilates system.

Important qualities in the Pilates system include dynamic movement, dynamic balance, dynamic placement, dynamic equilibrium. Movement is absolutely essential. If you lose your balance during an exercise, that's okay because your body and mind are searching. I don't think of this process as making a mistake; you're not doing anything wrong. Your body and mind are increasing their dynamic control of daily physical skills and preparing for action. That's all. In some ways, we find parallels in life. There are many times when we temporarily lose our emotional balance in life or we want to re-adjust our emotional balance to achieve certain goals or adapt to changing circumstances. We may fall, so to speak, but we learn and stand up again. We may change throughout life in one sense, but we keep our essence. Just keep moving, look forward, and stay hopeful while enjoying the pleasures of family, friends, and good work.

Pilates prepares you for those times when you don't feel on top of the world. This often occurs after a serious physical injury. In the aftermath, vulnerability and frustration rear their ugly heads. Recently I jumped over a campfire to practice a gymnastic somersault, and I broke my shoulder. I struggled to learn, adapt, and grow beyond that experience. By staying positive, you can increase awareness, learn new safe ways of moving, and help others develop these skills. Mistakes and accidents are opportunities to make you more insightful, more self-aware. Pilates is strongly connected with self-empowerment, preparing you for difficult times and physical challenges. Life is challenging, so we have to be mentally and physically tough. There is no way around it. We have to fight; we have to go into battle; we have to use weapons of survival. Joe Pilates was this way. Look at archival footage of him demonstrating his exercises. He was physically powerful with a strong mind. It's important to understand that his original system of Contrology will keep us strong and adaptable. Even when people don't take care of their bodies or their health in reasonable ways, it's never too late to invest time and effort. As human beings, we live, work, have babies, and have so many other responsibilities. Suddenly, 10-15 years pass; we look in the mirror and say, "Oh, I have a body that doesn't feel good. I'm tired, overweight. I have problems with my liver or it's difficult to twist my back, turn my head, and look behind me."

I have had challenges in my life. Professional acting has been my passion, yet it's a tough business. There are times when you don't have good contracts or sustainable work. This situation can be difficult, resulting in disappointment. When I found Classical Pilates, it provided me with a way to remain resilient in the face of difficulty. I like working with my body and my mind; I like to be challenged every day. The body is different every day; you feel things differently, but you must always find a way to establish mental control. Your mind is the boss.

Although I'm still a professional actor, I only choose the roles that are best for me. This is empowering. It is also great because I love teaching and have my own studio, Gen Pilates. It stands for Genetic. There are two reasons for this name: (1) I began learning The Work from my brothers Juan Pablo Ruiz and Juan Gabriel Ruiz; and (2) the Traditional Pilates system begins from such a deep place in my being that it feels bio-evolutionary or genetic! So, I can do The Work I love and help others improve their health and their strengths. My life has dynamic balance now. It's important to feel the sense of achievement that comes from cultivating health and wellness. Joe Pilates called it Contrology or the art of control—to be mentally disciplined and in charge of your own body. Many people don't live in their own bodies; it's strange but commonplace. I feel a strong sense of reward and satisfaction when I help students achieve the bodies and minds they want. To see a client living in his body with good energy, health, mental alertness and well-being is exciting! They are living up to their full potential; they go to work with more vitality; they ride a bicycle or walk with better coordination; they have positive mental attitudes; and they begin to smile more frequently. And when you smile, the world smiles with you.

About Juan:

Juan "Negro" Luis Ruiz Seckel began training in Classical Pilates during 2007 with professionals who were trained and certified by Romana Kryzanowska. Throughout the years, Negro has studied with Dorothee VandeWalle, Kathryn Ross-Nash, Peter Fiasca, Ilaria Cavagna, Jerome Weinberg and other experienced teachers. During 2014-2015 Negro continued rigorous in-depth study with Kathi Ross-Nash and successfully completed the Pilates Professional Advanced Teacher Training program. Since 2014 Negro has regularly traveled to New York City to train with professionals who preserve the values and teachings of Joe Pilates. Negro established his own training center called Gen Pilates (www.GenPilates.cl) and shares his knowledge with a wide variety of clients, as well as fellow professionals by teaching lessons and workshops. During 2016 Negro organized and produced the international educational event, which hosted Jerome Weinberg in Santiago de Chile.

Transformation Through Pilates

By Martt Lawrence

> ***...quickly noticing changes in his body and his athletic performance.***

Because it's our job as Pilates instructors to transform clients, we don't expect to be transformed by them. But often we are. It's no surprise that it happens in the same way that we change their bodies, which is to say that it happens gradually over time. I know, because it happened to me. The Work transformed my client's life, Jon, and he, in turn, changed my life.

A new male client in my studio recently commented that despite his years as an athlete, Pilates was the hardest physical activity he's ever done. I suspect that he's not the only man who has come to that conclusion. Aside from the practical aspects of male versus female progression through The Method, teaching Pilates to men is different than teaching women because, as a teacher, you can ride a fine line between challenging and humiliating men. This can sometimes be particularly tricky when a female instructor trains a male client.

There are myriad reasons why men won't even attempt Pilates. Often their reluctance is based on the simple misconception that Pilates is easy. Those who are familiar with the history of Pilates know that these misunderstandings are far from the truth. I suspect that Joe himself would roll over in his grave at the mere suggestion that The Work he created is easy or feminine. In my experience, many men willing to give Pilates a go come into the studio because of an injury or because Pilates is recommended to them by a friend, physical therapist, or doctor. Other men are drawn to Pilates because of their partners or wives. If they do try it, men are quite often surprised when they discover that Pilates is fun and challenging, as well as therapeutic for their injuries and complementary to their other activities.

As Pilates instructors, we set out to help people discover their bodies, their breath, critical core strength, and, subsequently, a better sense of themselves. Many of our clients make big strides over time, but at first we are very satisfied with hearing about the little things that have changed for them since they started taking Pilates. They often report being more comfortable in their own skin, their clothes finally fit them well again, and other people notice they are standing taller. It is our job to transform clients, and through the experience of doing Pilates ourselves, we know that The Method works.

My tale of transformation begins in the mid-nineties. I was a newly certified Pilates Instructor of 22, launching my career just before the dot-com industry became synonymous with Silicon Valley. I was passionate about The Work and hungry to teach. I was hungry in general, because I'd only just finished my apprenticeship, so when Jon walked into the studio, I was determined to make a good connection and introduce him to the wonders of Pilates. Jon, on the other hand, had only observed Pilates through our storefront window. Before he took his lesson, I asked him about his first impression of Pilates. He laughed, "I saw you all in there when I was walking by and thought, *What are they doing? That looks absolutely bizarre.*

When Jon and his muscles first shuffled into the studio, he was wearing long board shorts, a T-shirt, sandals, and a baseball cap, even though it was December. A 200-pound, muscle-bound, thirtysomething lawyer, Jon's idea of fun was being dropped from a helicopter onto a mountain peak, skiing down its steepest slope. He inquired about Pilates on the recommendation of a doctor who thought it would alleviate his chronic back pain. When we started our work together, he approached Pilates with some skepticism, planting a seed of doubt in my mind that he would be a good student. However, knowing that Jon was an athlete, I knew he had an inherent respect for the consistency of learning a skill. I hoped this would encourage him to stick with our work long enough to understand and feel its benefits.

In my first lesson with Jon, I learned a valuable lesson; it's easy to teach someone whose body is just like yours, but much harder to relate to a body very different from your own. Having never worked with anyone who had a stature like Jon's, the boundaries of my own skill level were tested, and I had to rethink my expectations for a beginner like him. In Footwork, he could not straighten his legs. It was as if they had never straightened completely before! His Hundred looked like a blowfish gasping for air! When we moved to the Mat, his lack of coordination seemed to defy all the ways in which I had been trained to work with bodies. He was so tight that lying on his back and pulling his knees into his chest proved impossible.

Though I didn't know it at the time, I came close to completely overstepping the humiliation line in my first session with him, a fact he reminded me of recently. "I don't know if you remember this," he said, "but you told me, 'You have a lot of superficial muscle. I don't know how this will go, but let's try it.'" He continued, "That's how we got started, and I felt quite flattered that I looked so muscular, but I could immediately tell I was not the standard candidate for Pilates."

Despite this rocky start, Jon made steady progress, quickly noticing changes in his body and his athletic performance, "I say this without wanting to sound like a commercial, but within a few weeks of starting the program, I noticed big gains in other things like skiing and working out at the gym." And these changes were enough to commit him to the system: "I remember working with you for about a month or two and then going away for a couple months. I continued to do some of the Mat work you taught me while I was away on this big ski trip. It helped stabilize my back, and assuage my fear of having my back blow out in the wilderness of Canada. I was so appreciative of what you were teaching me. That was the very beginning. I remember it vividly."

I doubt that Jon ever considered his bulk as a detriment. Fortunately, he was open to discovering the possibilities of strength with flexibility. Being a good-natured kind of guy, laughter became a huge part of our client/trainer relationship. Humor is helpful when training anyone, but it is particularly helpful in training men because it can lighten those potentially awkward moments when they are struggling with the flexibility challenges that Pilates brings. Jon was generally in good spirits when he came in, and it was because of this that we had a lot of fun with The Work. He enjoyed finding ways of renaming the exercises so that he could relate better to them. Pulling Straps became Surfing, Long Stretch became Hang Gliding, Side Splits became Skate Practice. These are images I still use today. They are more effective with men, giving them movements they can relate to or easily imagine.

Jon's bulk was such that one of his thighs was equal to both of mine. After working on exercises like Double Leg Kick, I often had to help him stretch. "I remember one time," he said, "You were trying to get me to be more flexible, and I was really struggling. You were very light, and you jumped on me to get me to stretch more. That was very funny, and it worked!" When I knelt down, putting all my weight on his hindquarters to get him into the rest position, we both cracked up at the disparity in our body types—he with his muscles and mass and I with my slight dancer's body. It just goes to show you that if you hit the right balance, clients will have fun while improving their bodies, and you'll keep them coming back for more.

Jon's practice of Pilates quickly and significantly minimized the frequency of his back episodes. One day, he was completely lopsided when he walked into the studio, his torso shifted significantly to the right, his hips and legs trailing on the left. My eyes bugged out of their sockets in amazement. Here was a man I knew to be relatively symmetrical in the musculature of his back, but in that moment he looked like someone with severe scoliosis. Jon recalled this particular occasion; "I was all twisted up, and you were so concerned about me. You said you didn't think we should do Pilates, but I insisted. I thought, worst case scenario, it would just look really funny! We both laughed at how contorted I was, but I immediately started to feel better, and we had a great time working through some physical discomfort and challenge in that session."

Because Jon had dealt with the problem in the past, he knew that the issue would resolve itself in a matter of days. We agreed that he should stay far away from doctors when he was in that condition, since they would immediately deem him a candidate for emergency surgery. As for me, I simply did my best to train him, my foremost goal just keeping him out of pain. To my surprise, he returned the following week looking and feeling normal, his spine back in alignment.

Jon slowly progressed from basic to intermediate, and eventually I was able to introduce advanced work. For him, the most appealing aspect of Pilates was the immediate, tangible benefits. Jon remarked, "I also responded immediately to how quickly you can progress. Whether you are great at it right away or whether you are terrible at it, you see very quickly that you are improving. That's a very engaging aspect of The Work. And, I felt better." It was gratifying to hear Jon's reports about skiing without pain, how he "dialed in," as he called it, to the intended muscles needed while surfing, all due to his Pilates training. In his words, "Like any craft, if you dedicate yourself to it with any consistency and just keep showing up, great stuff happens."

After one of our sessions, Jon announced that the dot-com company he worked for was treating him quite well financially, and he would give me a loan if I ever wanted to open my own business. He repeated this offer nearly every week. Though I was flattered, it took me years to mentally prepare for that possibility and to spin the idea into a reality. As I gradually gave him the confidence to trust his body, he gave me the confidence to open my own studio.

Jon first began training with me in 1996, and in 2005 he wrote me a check that enabled me to follow my professional dreams. "I was inspired by your dedication to Pilates and the people that you work with," Jon recalled. "And so I thought, if I can help you pursue your dreams and bring this good energy into the world, it's a privilege for me to be part of that."

After he explained the amortization schedule and the contract of repayment, he told me bluntly, "Martt, if something happens, and you can't pay me back, I don't care." This was what I needed to move forward without getting too stressed about the financial burden. His loan expanded my potential in the world, and his generosity gave me the courage to make my dream a reality. I would do everything I could to make sure I paid him back. Every cent.

Working with Jon over the years, I learned how to adapt my teaching skills for men. There were no jock lawyers at the arts schools I had attended or the dance companies with whom I had performed. He was a different breed. But I learned how to teach him, and his body was transformed by The Method. Of The Work, Jon said "Not only did it help my confidence as an athlete, but it was a great experience to try something so completely foreign, something I never would have considered. Pilates really helped me physically. My body felt completely different after doing it for a couple years."

Pilates transformed Jon, and in turn, his generosity transformed my life. Thanks to the backing of one of my earliest, most colorful and determined students, I founded The Pilates Center of San Francisco in 2006. My work continues daily as I support my clients, teachers, and apprentices in their own transformations.

About Martt:

The Pilates Center of San Francisco was opened in January of 2006 when owner Martt Lawrence seized an opportunity to make an impact on the dance community she knew and loved. After instructing the dancers at the San Francisco Ballet for five years, she was chosen by Brenda Way at ODC to run her own studio inside the commons.

Now in her twentieth year of teaching Pilates, Martt has studied with the best classical teachers in the industry including Romana Kryzanowska, Jay Grimes, Peter Fiasca, Kathryn Ross-Nash, Carol Appel, and most consistently with Dorothee VandeWalle, whom she has been mentored by since 2005.

Rehabilitation, Resiliance, and Vitality

By Kerry De Vivo and Erik Fridley

...clear connections as to how students can include their Pilates skills in other physical activities.

KERRY: Erik and I first met sailing. At the time, he was also an avid rugby player. Despite his active lifestyle and relative youth, he suffered from back pain. At a mutual friend's house one day, he began telling me about his discomfort. Although he was in his late 20s, back pain already affected his athletic performance. "You should try Pilates," I suggested. "You probably need to stretch your muscles, decompress your vertebrae, and increase core muscle strength." This piqued Erik's interest. But I didn't have to do much selling of Pilates; anything that minimized pain appealed to him. He understood that flexibility wasn't his forte, and I explained that Pilates addressed this issue. I knew the work would benefit him, so I invited him to Excel Pilates to train with apprentice teachers. This was an excellent, cost-free, and immediate way to start practicing the Traditional Method.

ERIK: During that time, I had herniated discs in my back that eventually required surgery. In addition, I had a rugby injury, a strained right quadriceps, which was the result of a singular event. I must have pulled this muscle because it was extremely tight. That's when Kerry introduced me to Pilates. The emphasis of training was pain management to reduce symptoms in my back. Sitting was very difficult. I tried to manage the pain myself by stretching, even running, but to no avail. Neither chiropractic nor physical therapy treatments were effective either. Yet when I started Pilates, the pain relief was almost immediate. Although I stopped playing rugby for half of the full season, I returned for a relatively short period of time, but my body could no longer excel at high levels in that kind of sport. The physical intensity—muscular abuse—of the game was too much. My body needed to heal. And it appreciated Pilates for this, as well as conditioning. To balance my continued interest in a physically demanding activity, I increased the frequency of running, as Pilates improved my core strength and flexibility. I was fortunate to train in Pilates three to five times per week with apprentices.

It's been almost 13 years since that time. The pain is actually difficult to remember. But at the time my day-to-day existence was compromised. I could barely go to the office, and I couldn't sit in my chair or stand in a stationary position for any extended period of time. Co-workers often found me lying on the floor, stretching my back muscles. After starting Pilates, however, I literally found that point of release where I could alleviate the sciatic pain radiating down my legs and around the front of my body. The beneficial effects of Pilates were almost immediate. My quality of life improved so much that I could actually sit in the car for extended periods of time and travel for family or work trips.

Engaging my abdominals and scoop-lifting all the time, even sitting in my car, reduced back discomfort. Pilates muscle action eliminated pain in my back, legs, feet, abdominals, and my entire body. The work didn't just strengthen my back and core; it aligned my body, stretching and lengthening to the point where I could feel and notice significantly improved posture. If I were sitting incorrectly at my desk, if I hunched forward, that negatively affected my back, and I immediately experienced pain. But if I scooped and sat tall, the pain dissipated.

For nearly four years, I studied 2-3 times a week at an advanced level. Kerry rarely taught me, though, because she had so many existing clients to attend to. Once in a while we trained together, and on those occasions she explained elements of the system as we practiced the exercises. Students or clients sometimes fail to understand that the Traditional Pilates system has pace. There's a dynamic to each exercise, a timing of transition to each successive exercise; if you wait too long or you move too fast, the workout isn't cohesive. So it means you have to have the proper pace. When you're training with somebody like Kerry, you're kept on a rhythm. That's how The Work was meant to be taught; that's how you get the most out of Pilates. I learned these concepts from her. When the apprentices trained me, sometimes I got ahead of them during the lesson. Then they began to understand my timing.

During this time, there were two big changes in my life: the transition away from rugby and an increased commitment to sailing, which included local and international competitions. In sailing, my biggest improvement was balance. It was a powerful change for me to engage my entire body; sailboats constantly move through linear motion (heave, sway, surge) and rotation (pitch, roll, yaw), tilting, turning and tipping while the crew works in every position. Pilates enabled me to move more quickly on the sailboat. It gave me better stability and coordination. Everyone called me a monkey! I developed more agility, stamina and strength, climbing the mast without a rope, as if it were a coconut tree!

Balance is important on larger boats, like mine, as well as smaller boats. When it's just a two-man boat, it's best to engage 100% of your core muscles just to keep the boat level. With my back problems, some people said, "You're nuts." But they didn't understand how I safely exerted my body because of Pilates. The biggest challenge was managing pain while sustaining enough core strength to sail competitively without compromising my back. In time, I returned to soccer, which helped my overall balance, speed, and flexibility. When I play soccer, most often I'm the only team member stretching before and after the game. Sometimes when I'm in a rush, I just practice the Pilates Series of Five or a quick intermediate Pilates Mat workout; they both warm up my body and give me good flexibility; it doesn't take that long—five or ten minutes.

KERRY: Pilates gives Erik agility and flexibility; in turn, these qualities provide foundational support for the intense strength demands of rugby. A challenging sport like this requires force and strength. Pilates reveals what I call "true valuable strength." Agility and flexibility are necessary but not sufficient conditions; however, these "vehicles of strength" are underused in sports training.

ERIK: The older you get, the less physically efficient you become, so it's important to intelligently condition and train the body. Traditional Pilates work provides technique that improves muscular efficiency, energy efficiency, and mental efficiency. Before I studied Pilates, I expended a great deal of energy—too much energy—on the field just with tackles, running, pacing, and supporting my body. When I learned Pilates, I could control my body with optimum levels of physical and mental energy. As a result of increased efficiency, I had more stamina and strength during the game. My body became more intelligent, too, because I initiated all movement from core Powerhouse muscles, and I better understood the center of gravity, dynamic balance, precision, and coordination.

Many people support their torsos primarily with back muscles; they might think, *I have good posture.* Yet if they're not using core muscles (abdominals, inner thighs, gluteals), the back muscles frequently absorb too much weight load. As a result, there is more likelihood of muscle strain. Getting in and out of the car, moving a box, cleaning the house, picking up groceries, carrying your kids. All of these activities require balanced muscle work for good posture and effective use of your body. This is the most amazing benefit of Pilates.

Many people say, "Oh, I do Pilates," but all too often they don't understand the depth of The Work. I know I didn't at first. It's really a method of Contrology, as Joe Pilates wrote in his books—the technique of optimally controlling your body by identifying and working those small muscle groups to support and guide larger muscle groups. As soon as you discover how to properly recruit the right muscles, it's like, wow! Everything changes for the better. Nothing illustrates this principle better than the Pull-Up exercise on the Wunda Chair. When you first attempt this exercise, you stand on the pedal and it doesn't move. When you find how and where to engage core muscles, suddenly the pedal naturally rises. It's a huge accomplishment for anyone. For me, lifting the pedal was a challenge because I'm not the most flexible person. Of course, you can cheat by leaning the body too far forward. But good teachers push your shoulders back to sustain correct alignment and engage the proper muscles.

Practicing Contrology gives you a "reset button" for your brain. I incorporated Pilates as a type of stress relief or mental decompression: focusing, concentrating, and being present during each exercise, each movement, making sure that I practiced correctly. If I arrive at the studio experiencing work stress, a thousand thoughts running through my brain, as soon as I begin The Hundred, my mind is focused only on Pilates. The stress goes away; I can't even remember the 1,000 things I was thinking about until I re-engage with the world after my workout. In that way, Pilates is therapy for the mind, what Joe Pilates called mental conditioning.

KERRY: Erik is a much happier person when he does Pilates regularly. He is an extremely good student—hardworking, focused, open-minded, and coordinated. He readily understands verbal instruction and enjoys trying new ways of executing movement. Erik is really tuned in to his body, enabling him to connect different muscle groups into an organized whole. And he understands how Pilates builds on past abilities and strengths to meet current demands on the body.

Stress reduction is an important part of practicing Pilates. When you're moving, when you're mentally focused, the experience is extremely rewarding; life is good. All through my 20s and into my 30s, I rehearsed every day and performed frequently. Then life began to change; I had a job, a mortgage, a child; "me time" diminished. There was less time to play team sports like rugby or soccer or a group sport such as sailing. These activities became time commitments that, in this stage of life, weren't available without creating even more stress.

Pilates isn't a team sport, so it's just a matter of fitting it into your own schedule. It is a great way to stay conditioned, active, and skillful; as Joseph Pilates wrote in his books, The Work prepares you to safely and effectively accomplish daily activities, skilled sports, and unexpected movements. Erik is in such good shape that he recently participated in a 5K. If you train the right way, Pilates sustains your physical strength and skills even when you don't have time to participate in other skilled sports.

ERIK: Rugby encompasses a wide range of body types and sizes, whereas in soccer you typically don't see 285-pound, 6' 5" guys. On the rugby field, though, you may see a 135-pound winger as well as a 300-pound hook or frontman. Each of these body types adopts a different workout to stay in good physical shape and condition their bodies. Some of the bigger guys lift weights; they like the heavy work. But weight lifting in itself doesn't translate into improved overall conditioning or the ability to adequately stretch within an optimal range of motion for the game. Although the weight lifter might bench press 300 pounds, I get the same workout in Pilates without the strain, and I actually engage more muscles, lengthening and strengthening and increasing flexibility. I don't need to lift 300-pound weights because I do Pilates; I have the strength, the agility, the flexibility, and the speed to outperform any weight lifter.

If you have intelligent control of your body, you can accomplish both reasonable and remarkable skills. When I was studying Pilates regularly and playing rugby, the coach put me in the fullback position. The reason? I was able to chase down anybody on the field and make every tackle. It wasn't because I was the best player on the field; it was because I was more physically efficient than the person running toward me. And I was able to tackle properly; I could bring a 300-pound player to the ground and not get hurt.

When I don't have 50 minutes for a lesson, I do my own workout, which I named, Ten, Ten and Ten. I practice ten Pilates exercises for ten minutes around 10:00 PM. Then I go to bed. This workout is a great mental/physical reset, relieving the stress after a long day at work. It enables me to wind down and relax, so I get a good night's sleep. I have practiced Ten, Ten and Ten almost every night for years. If more men understood the benefits of Pilates, they would follow suit. Sadly, though, they have the impression that Pilates is for women. They just don't understand what a strong, vigorous workout it is.

KERRY: People say, "Oh, you teach Pilates. Is it like yoga? Martial arts? Swimming?" I always explain, "Pilates was an actual person who developed this discipline; it's unique and the only way to understand it is to experience it." When I started Pilates, I had played many sports - swimming, track and field, gymnastics, dance, basketball, everything! But no other discipline required me to use my body in the ways that Pilates does, and no other discipline offers the benefits of Pilates. When people are correctly taught the Pilates system, they really experience the value, but it's experiential like any sport. Of course I can describe the benefits, but until you physically experience them, you can't know. There are myriad misunderstandings, myths, and misconceptions about Pilates.

When I introduce Pilates to novices, I explain the apparatus in a way that enables them to better understand the system: "When you work with springs, you develop your body and your muscles like springs. They're strong, articulate, and flexible. You practice controlled movement using good concentration." For weight lifters or athletes who play high impact sports or other physical activities with repetitive actions, my approach is different. I ask what their goals are in the sport they play: "Do you want to develop or enhance certain physical skills? Do you want to become a lean, mean fighting machine?

Are you training to become a cheetah or a bull?" Then I integrate the clients' goals into their lessons—often without them knowing it—and periodically make a comment to deepen their understanding of The Work and develop visual-visceral connections.

Joe Pilates wrote that physical fitness requires excellent mental concentration; he also wrote about the uniform development of all muscle groups. Yet for a lot of people, the primary test of physical fitness is how well you fit into your jeans, the simple outline of your physique, your outer appearance. Of course these goals matter, but they should be the result of working the mind and body with deep intelligence, as Joe Pilates espoused and practiced. In this respect, there are some differences between men and women. As teachers, we can anticipate different typical gender-related motivations, although oftentimes these goals are based on life stages, not gender. Occasionally, I experience frustration and disappointment with client expectations and motivation for undertaking Pilates. These students unwittingly deprive themselves of experiencing the truly rich and transformative health benefits of Joe Pilates' work. The silver lining, though, is that just by being in the studio and learning the technique, they are working toward Joe Pilates' highest ideals! There is only one student whom I threatened, "If you use the word liposuction one more time here in the Pilates studio, you can't come back."

Pilates is about efficiency of movement, good mental concentration and the practice of fewer repetitions done at peak performance. Then you move on. Most men start Pilates with a different mentality, though. If an athletic man comes to the studio and doesn't feel maximum strenuous work bordering on pain, if he doesn't grunt and groan, or if he doesn't leave the studio dripping with sweat, he assumes he didn't get a good workout. So, as an instructor, it's important to be strict and demanding like Joe Pilates, but not push men to exhaustion and fatigue for their own sake. Believe me, when Pilates is taught correctly, men understand the challenges and work hard. Sometimes I give the Pull-Up exercise on the Wunda Chair or another exercise that makes them take stock of themselves and their limitations. A strong man in good physical condition will be frustrated when he can't do an exercise. Then I demonstrate it. When a slender 5' 2" woman can accomplish the exercise effortlessly, a man thinks, *I've got to be able to do this.* But no one can execute the Pull-Up without the right muscular connections; it takes time. Some people want to learn and others aren't ready yet. But it's a fascinating process for teachers, as clients learn new ways to work muscles.

For some people, Pilates prepares them for activities of daily living; for others, it is a means to physically and mentally accomplish the skilled sports they love; and for still others, it prevents injury and increases longevity. Some exercise enthusiasts get a high from running, but the weight-load impact on joints (ankles, knees, hips) causes biomechanical strain, putting them at risk for injury. In the over-40 soccer league, the most frequently asked question is, "What's the injury of the season?" I joke about it, but each year there's a commonly occurring injury among the players. What if more people practiced Pilates? They would have a proven system for injury prevention and improved athletic performance related to daily functional movement, recreational activity, and professional sports.

Overall, Americans could benefit from developing a better understanding of what it means to be physically fit. A large segment of the fitness industry firmly believes in pushing individuals to strenuous extremes where exhaustion and fatigue are primary goals. Joe Pilates absolutely disagreed with this approach; he wanted students to leave the studio energized, agile, strong, flexible, mentally focused, and in full control of their coordination to live healthy, productive lives. Traditional Pilates provides the best discipline for optimal physical and mental fitness. It's important to learn about your body, understand your body, manage your body so you can achieve varied daily activities with spontaneous zest and pleasure.

ERIK: There are a few aspects of Pilates that most people don't understand. When the system is taught correctly, it provides people with a "serious workout" because of the cardiovascular conditioning, the simultaneous stretching and strengthening with strong weight-bearing spring resistance, and the heightened mental alertness. As a result, I only need Pilates. There's no need to do several different workouts in a single day; there's no need to lift weights or use machines at a gym. In the Pilates studio, I get a "heavy workout" that meets all of my goals. Don't misunderstand. I'm not saying Pilates is the easy way out; it's not. It's actually the most difficult workout—if done well. Pilates, taught correctly and correctly learned, is hard; it's also the most efficient way of optimally training your body and mind. It keeps your life in control in order to live well with great energy. Furthermore, you feel good after the workout. You think, *Wow, that was a fantastic workout and my mind is clear. Now I'm ready to tackle any challenge.* I say tackle because there's a strong sense of physical and mental achievement after the workout. The system is extremely challenging, yet it's accessible to everyone.

KERRY: When someone studies Pilates, I never suggest they abandon any other physical activity they enjoy. People run or practice weight training or use the elliptical machine. They often confess, "I like doing these things, but I feel pain." So I respond, "Let's transfer this information to Pilates." One student with severe scoliosis had an epiphany during the Stomach Massage exercise. I knew she included Leg Press exercises in her weight training routine, so I asked her to look closely at the action in Stomach Massage. "You know the core muscles are driving this exercise. So what's the difference between this and Leg Press at the gym?" "Right, nothing," she responded. Expounding, I reminded her, "You don't have to hurt your back doing Leg Press if you initiate the movement from your Powerhouse."

My role teaching Traditional Pilates includes helping people understand how to work their bodies correctly, safely, strongly, flexibly. And I make clear connections as to how students can include their Pilates skills in other physical activities. Individuals in their 40s, 50s, and 60s feel younger as a result of the changes in their bodies. They want to feel structure, strength, flexibility, support, and agility in all physical activities.

Long ago, I taught a young football player on the University of Maryland team. This man went on to play professionally in the NFL. One day during a Pilates lesson, he remarked, "Man, this is so much harder than practice; I have to really pay attention all the time." To study Pilates well, you must develop concentration, because the system is an all-encompassing workout.

ERIK: Sadly, there is a flip side to what Kerry is describing. With the intention of increasing cardio fitness, you can take spinning class for an hour in a body position where your shoulders are strained and potentially injured. But I can get the same cardio workout in Pilates with my shoulders in proper position, my wrists relaxed, my neck and back working well and my entire body in optimal placement with perfect alignment. Unfortunately, many people think about physical exercise in this way: *Oh, I've got to be spinning for an hour to get a cardio workout, then I have to lift weights to get strong, then I have to stretch to get flexible, and so on.* Before you realize the time investment, you've worked out for six hours! Now you're exhausted and upset because there's no time to attend to your professional work! I'm not looking for the easy way out by simply reducing workout time to a 50-minute Pilates lesson. The fact is that anyone can accomplish so much more in Traditional Pilates compared to their current workouts. And as a bonus, everything you've worked for in Pilates can be applied to vigorous athletics or everyday movement.

When I started doing Pilates at 29, I was physically very active in sports. For three to five years I regularly trained in Pilates. My body was in a great place: it was achieving peak performance, and I enjoyed great dynamic balance. At age 33, I was diagnosed with cancer. Looking back on that situation, if I had not been in excellent physical condition, the effects of chemotherapy would have been different. I continued to work out during treatments, although not as frequently. Pilates was critical in helping me sustain a full and positive life when I was being beaten down, so to speak, by all the chemicals and drugs. The mental aspect was important, too. You just don't know what life is going to bring you. One day I was doing great, enjoying a visit with the family for Easter. Then just prior to church, I found a lump; it was that quick. Yet Pilates had prepared my body and mind to be resilient under any circumstance. This is a main theme in Joe Pilates' writings. Having the confidence that your body and mind are sufficiently well-conditioned to endure cancer is powerful. In the Pilates system you have to mentally dig deep in all workouts to make it work and to get something out of it. Having cancer, it was important that I really dig deep to maintain optimism. Thirty days after my chemotherapy was complete, I ran a 10 kilometer race. Pilates had a profoundly positive impact on my life, and it still does. Whether you have a serious illness, or you're as healthy as an ox, I highly recommend it.

About Kerry:

Kerry De Vivo began studying Pilates in 1986 with Steve Giordano at SUNY Purchase. She received her Pilates certification in 1995 with master teacher Romana Kryzanowska and went on to co-found Excel Movement Studios in Washington, DC. In 2002, she co-founded Excel Pilates in Annapolis.

Effortless Power

By Allan Nathan

...super jocks are struck by the relaxed power of my movements.

I am an athlete. Driven to challenge myself physically and mentally, I relish testing the limits of my strength, stamina and determination. As far back I can remember, the sports arena has been my domain. Throughout elementary and high school, I pursued excellence on the basketball court. When I graduated from college, I began a long journey into martial arts. My first teacher was Tadashi Nakamura, a prolific author, founder of the World Seidō Karate Organization and one of the foremost Japanese karate instructors in the world.

Seidō is physically challenging, but for Nakamura, it encompasses much more than fighting ability. Ideally, it develops an individual physically, spiritually and morally. However, like many novices in the martial arts, I disregarded its Zen-like aspect and pushed myself physically, sometimes beyond my limits. Before long, I graduated to more challenging styles, placing increasingly more stress on my body. The breaking point came when I expanded my repertoire to include one of the most demanding martial arts moves. Repeatedly executing shin kicks on a heavy bag, I put tremendous pressure on my lumbar spine. Not surprisingly, I herniated L4 and L5 disks.

By the time I reached the physical therapist, I could no longer perform a full split. In fact, I could barely bend forward more than three inches. The protective mechanisms of my body had activated to prevent me from doing further damage to my already savaged body. When my therapist learned that I practiced Brazilian jiu-jitsu, she suggested, “Perhaps you want to re-think that, and try Pilates.” Although at the time I was studying yoga, she was adamant—Pilates.

Under the guidance of Romana-certified trainer Tonka Cascais in Ft. Lauderdale, Florida, slowly but surely, I regained my strength and flexibility. At first I didn’t really grasp the concept of Pilates. It was more of a physical practice for me. But that was enough to keep me coming back. Eventually, I moved to New York, studying at True Pilates. It was then that I really began to understand Pilates as more than merely a physical practice.

And I began to see the parallel between the principles of Pilates and the Japanese and Zen Buddhist approach to martial arts; both stressed centering, concentration, control, breath and flow. What was missing from the tenets of martial arts, however, was precision, a crucial factor in protecting the body. To become extremely efficient, extremely powerful, you can't just rely on your physicality—muscles and tendons. If you don't have structural integrity within the body, you're always going to be just muscling through movements. And that's what led me to a herniated disk.

My lack of structural integrity was painfully evident in those early Pilates sessions. As one of the biggest clients in the studio, I felt like a bull in a china shop. First of all, the ratio of female to male at the studio was at least 10:1. And these lithe but powerful women were doing things that in my wildest dreams I couldn't imagine doing at that time. What really impressed me, though, was the degree to which it appeared to be effortless. That's what I had been seeking all along. I mean, let's face it. How long can you retain your physical strength and vigor? At some point you have to bend, learn how to yield in life. If you just meet opposition head-on continually, you set yourself up for injury.

Not one knows that better than I. You see, I suffer from "big man's syndrome." While this disease isn't listed in any medical text book, all you have to do is walk into any gym to see numerous examples of this testosterone-based disorder. At 6'4", 220 pounds, when I exert force against any external object, I am used to muscling my way through it. But you can't do that in Pilates because you're not really working against an external force. Being larger than everyone else, I was used to moving heavier loads. And I have longer levers! So I had to learn to integrate the whole body as one unit, as opposed to initiating from the extremities and moving each part segmentally.

When you move from your Center there is less stress on your joints and you are far more powerful. And what man isn't looking to produce more power and force? What is unique in the Pilates system is what I call "effortless power." You can produce 90% of the force that you would if you were just using pure physical strength. But you only use 50% to 60% of the energy, producing a level of force in a relaxed, effortless manner by expending a fraction of the energy. So you give up 10% of the power, but you're only using half of the energy. Suddenly your golf swing is more powerful, your forehand is stronger, you jump higher, all with less strain on your joints. In fact, it improves any athletic performance.

But this concept of moving from The Center is not new. Kinesiology, biomechanics, anatomy trains and muscle fascia theory stress proper body mechanics. And it is a cornerstone of martial arts. In Chinese Quigong, it is the Dantian. In Japanese, it is called hara, referring to the energy center located two or three inches beneath the navel. But Pilates does it comprehensively and simply. It addresses alignment from head to toe, starting from your feet, which provide the foundation, integrating every part of your body with the Powerhouse.

At the same time that I started my training in Pilates, I began dabbling in what is called the "softer" martial arts, which are more spiritual and less purely physical activity. Under the guidance of William C. C. Chen, I learned T'ai Chi. Chen first introduced me to the concept of internal power. To improve my practice, I actually had to take two steps back and let things go. By absorbing or yielding to the energy of an attack instead of opposing it with sheer force, one can neutralize it. This means that an extremely strong individual cannot just rely on his strength. He has to become soft. In order to have softness, he needs a degree of hardness. They work hand in hand to develop a more internal practice. At the time, I thought I grasped the concept of internal power and softness espoused in martial arts, but it was Pilates that taught me the true essence of effortless power.

Not only was Pilates the epitome of effortless power, but its spiritual component was attainable, almost tangible, unlike the mysterious mystical concept of T'ai Chi, a somewhat nebulous ability to project one's "life force." And in Pilates, if you worked hard enough, listened, focused, concentrated, controlled your movements and worked with the breath, the internal power appeared to be within reach. Granted, that could take two years, five years, but the beauty of Pilates is it's about the journey, not the destination. Reveling in the progress you make executing an exercise on different apparatus. Reflecting on movements you cannot perform, moving on and then suddenly accomplishing them. That's why I fell in love with Pilates and how I finally understood internal power.

But Pilates fascinated me in another way, as well. In my previous life, I was the head trader of equity derivatives at a major investment bank. Although it was an exciting business, it certainly had its pitfalls. Everyone knows about the misappropriations, the Bernie Madoffs, the unscrupulous people who lie, cheat, and steal for the almighty dollar. That's what I was up against every day of my life. How could I be sure what trades to take? Only through sufficient research and risk assessment could I avoid going the way of the dinosaur.

In trading there's a philosophy that people are based on one of two emotions, either fear or greed. And I'm a fear-based individual, motivating me to up the ante on research. These habits carried over to Pilates. I never take things at face value, preferring instead to do my research. Because Joe wrote something, I'll do it; but I'm going to try to understand why it works, how it works, what's behind it. In this way, the physical practice led to more of an intellectual practice. I began to read books on kinesiology, biomechanics. I even called Stuart McGill, author, professor and Director of the Spine Biomechanics Laboratory at the University of Waterloo. "Why does this work? What is the advantage of this?" I inquired. And then I began to see the logic behind the principles Joe developed. Everything I read or heard from these experts explained and confirmed the genius of Pilates. My scientific brain craved facts, as so much of Pilates training is qualitative. Through intensive study and years of teaching so many different bodies, teachers develop a more instinctive understanding of what the human body responds to and what it doesn't. Unlike these naturally gifted, instinctive teachers, I needed to understand WHY it worked. And now I began to see it as more than an art. Now I saw the science behind it. Hungry for more, I took basic physics and elementary biomechanics.

It's not that I didn't have faith in The Method. I knew it worked. When I injured my back and I couldn't move, I went to physical therapy. Then I went to Pilates. And it was there I got better. The Work was so much more developed, advanced, well thought out than the physical therapy protocol I received that I knew there had to be something behind it.

And the fact that I struggled to master The Work helped my teaching. Sometimes teachers who are naturally gifted, having studied ballet all their lives, don't struggle the way a man my size does. By persevering, working through each level, each step to eventually conquer the advanced repertoire, I discovered what it meant to work through physical limitations. That made me a more compassionate teacher. And understanding biomechanics/kinesiology was just a guide.

The science of movement enabled me to comprehend what these naturally gifted teachers already knew. I couldn't just muscle my way through each movement, especially at the advanced level. But understanding about levers, resistance arms, torque, and, more importantly, the concept that total tension doesn't always work, I could work more efficiently. Sometimes you have to actually let go at the same time while engaging. And really that comes down to the agonist/antagonist muscle structure, learning that if you don't release the antagonist, you're working against yourself. It's really a little dance. Sometimes you have to stabilize a little bit better or you have to learn how to work with the breath better. The best teachers will teach you that.

To see the genius in Joe's system, you just have to read, "To Keep in Shape: Act Like An Animal" in Sports Illustrated, February 12, 1962. A true artist takes the chaos around him and systematizes it in a certain way, making order out of chaos, much the way I did as a trader. Joe's genius, aside from being an inventor and a visionary, is the way he systematized his method. Anyone can work within that system. If you put your mind to it, you can become an excellent teacher, whether your focus is fitness or rehabilitation. And within that systematized framework, every day you learn, picking up another piece of the puzzle.

Despite the genius of The Work, men just don't gravitate toward Pilates. I was one of those guys who believed it was an art that most fit, very athletic men really didn't need. I didn't see a purpose for it and didn't understand it. Joe alluded to it in his '62 article: "Americans! They want to go 600 miles an hour, and they don't know how to walk! Look at them in the street. Bent over." We're so goal driven that sometimes we don't understand the process of getting to that goal.

And Pilates has a stigma that it's predominantly a female art. Yet The Method was originally developed for men – boxers. If you look at some of the male practitioners, it's really incredible what they can do. Part of the problem is they do it so unobtrusively, so effortlessly. Unlike the testosterone driven workout of the muscle head, there is no breath holding, no bulging neck veins, no grunting. Thus, we assume it's not an exercise regimen that generates tremendous power. So how does one convert the heathens?

Converting a healthy guy, one who has no injuries, is the challenge. First, you must get his attention. A demonstration of something I know the other person can't do is usually all it takes. When I'm working out, particularly in a hardcore, weightlifting gym, people notice, especially men. They don't associate my workout with Pilates because they don't know it's Pilates. However, they do notice the flexibility, the control, and the strength underlying the movements. Invariably, they ask what I'm doing, especially if it involves flexibility. Most guys over 30 are lucky if they can pick up a piece of paper off the floor, so increasing their flexibility is important. But they also relate to the strength and control. When I kick or punch a heavy bag, these super jocks are struck by the relaxed power of my movements. Once I tell them it's Pilates, all of a sudden a little bell goes off. As soon as I see that recognition in their eyes, I seize the moment: "Why don't you train with me on Tuesday and Thursday at 6 PM?" I bring them into the fold.

Until they see a male practitioner, they just won't change their perspective on the art. It's difficult for them, as it was for me, to abandon the purely male energy, the yang in weightlifting. Pilates, with its lower resistance and reduced repetitions, provides a kind of yin/yang balance. Instead of fatiguing the muscles, leaving you exhausted, it energizes you, making your body feel good. And once they've experienced this, they rarely leave. My "ah-ha" moment was when I saw Kathi Ross-Nash and Jerome Weinberg executing super-advanced moves on the Cadillac and Reformer. They moved with such power and grace. I was hooked.

And once these weightlifters are hooked, they are the best ambassadors for Pilates. As they gain control and flexibility, they become more enthusiastic, spreading the word. Before long, the personal trainers, conditioning coaches and aerobics instructors notice the changes in physique and power, curious to learn more. In this way, the gym is the best source for potential Pilates clients.

No sales pitch is needed. When it comes to the magic of effortless power, seeing is believing!

About Allan:

Among his many achievements, Allan's career includes working as Managing Director and Head Trader of Equity Derivatives at two Wall Street investment banks, Nomura Securities as well as Smith Barney. Allan achieved his Third Degree Black Belt in Seido Karate under Kaicho Tadashi Nakamura who represented Seido Karate in Japan. In addition, Allan studied Tai Chi Chuan for 10 years under Grandmaster William Chi-Cheng Chen. Allan was the owner and director of Dojo Pilates in Sag Harbor, New York. Allan is currently living in Burlington, Vermont, and he is coaching boys' basketball at the Lake Champlain Waldorf School. Allan plans to establish a Pilates and bodyweight conditioning studio in Vermont with Classical Pilates as well as Tai Chi Chuan and the effortless power work of William C. C. Chen.

Pilates and Men

By Richard Rossiter

> ***...Joe wanted everyone to practice Contrology, and he did not care whether they were male or female.***

The Pilates Method of physical and mental conditioning is beset by an unfortunate and unfounded stereotype.

It can be observed that most men, who do not do Pilates, believe it is for women. They believe that the exercises are easy, or "stretchy," and do not require strength, nor do they build strength. Men play football, lift weights, work for a living, and drink beer, right? At least they watch football, think about lifting weights, work, and drink beer. Men who actually do Pilates, on the other hand, soon learn that The Work is quite challenging, requires great strength, and is certainly not just for women. So what is the source of this misunderstanding?

If we look at group photographs from Pilates conferences and workshops commonly posted on the Internet, we will see mostly women in attendance. We would get the same impression by walking into a Pilates studio almost anywhere in the world.

Joseph Pilates opened his original studio at 939 8th Avenue in Manhattan, three blocks south of Columbus Circle, in 1926. The studio, also known as the 939 Studio[1], was on the second floor and overlooked 8th Avenue. Joe and his life partner Clara (Anna Klara Zeuner) lived in a flat adjacent to the studio. Jay Grimes said, "Joe was a boxer. He didn't care about dancers. He opened his studio in deliberate proximity to Madison Square Garden,"[2] which in 1926 was just a few blocks away, at 50th Street and 8th Avenue.[3]

What was it like to work with Joseph Pilates?

Jay Grimes was a professional dancer who studied with Joseph Pilates in the mid-1960s and later with Joe's wife Clara. Jay said during a workshop at Brooke Siler's studio, NYC, "There is too much pampering and watering down of The Work these days. Joe just kicked your ass. He didn't care who you were."

Kathleen Stanford Grant (9 August 1921 to 27 May 2010) was a successful dancer and choreographer, but a knee injury and surgery interrupted her career. She was referred to Joseph Pilates by actress/singer Pearl Bailey in 1954 and began teaching for Carola Trier three years later. She was one of two students to receive a teaching certificate from Joseph Pilates through a program with the State University of New York. Kathleen said, "Pilates is hard. Joseph Pilates was a man and he created the exercises for men."[4]

Mary Bowen, a Jungian psychoanalyst, was a student at the 939 Studio from1959 to 1965.[5] Mary said, "Joe was in the body, very physical, driven, structured, German. They (Joe and Clara) were closed in emotionally, old world mentality, very professional, stern, drove clients to tears."

This is hardly a description of the Watercourse Way or the Feminine Principle in nature. So where did all the women come from?

Professional dancers came to Joe to get help with injuries and to strengthen their bodies. Many of these dancers were women, some of whom went on to open studios and to teach what they had learned from Joe and Clara. They, in turn, attracted more women (oftentimes dancers) to the Pilates Method, and so it has continued into present time.

Not everyone who came to Joe was a woman or a dancer, but almost. Bob Seed was a hockey player. John Winters was an organist. Both men studied long with Joe and became teachers at the 939 Studio. John Steele was an attorney, a student, and friend of the Pilates, who established the 939 Studio Corporation for Clara in February of 1970, and the Pilates Studio, Inc. in May of 1973.[6] Ralph Hollander, with the approval and assistance of Joseph Pilates, created The Pilates Foundation for Physical Fitness in 1965, a nonprofit corporation, which sought to promote and preserve the Pilates system of exercise.[7] Some of the men who came to work with Joe were dancers such as Ted Shawn, Barton Mumaw, Bruce King, Ron Fletcher, Robert Fitzgerald, and Jay Grimes. All but Shawn and Mumaw taught The Work throughout their lives. Jay Grimes is still teaching at his studio, Vintage Pilates, in West Los Angeles.

All things considered, most of those who came to the 939 Studio were dancers, and most of them were women. We cannot, in fact, separate the world of dance from Joseph Pilates. The man and his work just made sense to dancers. It is flatly ironic that Joseph Pilates said, "I don't like the dancers; they change my work."[8]

I attended the first meeting of the Pilates Method Alliance in South Beach, Florida, during spring of 2001. Most of the attendees were women. Kevin Bowen and Colleen Glenn collaborated to create a nonprofit organization dedicated to preserving the essence and value of the Pilates Method. They reached out and brought together Kathleen Grant, Ron Fletcher, Mary Bowen, and Lolita San Miguel. They also invited Romana Kryzanowska who declined the invitation. Each of these first generation teachers told their stories of how they came to meet Joe and Clara and what they were like. They gave candid impressions of the studio, The Work, the equipment, and told stories of the other students and teachers who were present at the 939 Studio. It was a unique event, a retelling of history, which would never happen in this way again.

It was mentioned in the presentations that Joseph Pilates met George Balanchine in the 1930s or '40s, that Balanchine had his dance company in the same building with Joe (939 8th Avenue), and that he oftentimes sent his dancers to work with Joe.[9] By 1946 Balanchine had established the School of American Ballet at the New York City Center, 131 West 55th Street, less than two blocks from Joe's studio. Balanchine's wife, Tanaquil Le Clercq, contracted polio in 1956; and she was sent to work with Joseph Pilates.[10] George Balanchine said, "Joseph Pilates is a genius of the body."[11]

Note: The term "Elder" has been widely applied to the students of Joseph and Clara Pilates who learned The Work at the 939 Studio and who taught The Work, there and elsewhere, during and after the lives of Joe and Clara. A comprehensive list of the Elders or first generation teachers must include Robert Fitzgerald, Ron Fletcher, Jay Grimes, Bruce King, Bob Seed, and Jonathan Winters (of the men); and Romana Kryzanowska. Naja Corey, Eve Gentry, Kathleen Grant, Hannah Sakmerda, Lolita San Miguel, Marry Bowen and Carola Trier (of the women). Of these, only Jay Grimes, Lolita San Miguel, and Mary Bowen are known to be alive.

Joe established a second studio at the Henri Bendel department store in 1965. Naja Corey, who was trained at the 939 Studio, taught at Bendel's from 1967 to 1972, when Kathleen Grant took over and ran the studio until its closure in 1988.[12] Bendel's was, and still is, an upscale women's specialty store at 712 Fifth Avenue, three blocks east of the 939 Studio. This was another of Joe's ventures destined to attract women (and not men) to the Pilates Method.

Joe and Clara purchased a "weekend property" in Becket, Massachusetts, consisting of more than 50 acres with a house on a small lake.[13] The property was within walking distance of a dance retreat called Jacob's Pillow, which began as a farm in 1790 on a mountain between Boston, Massachusetts, and Albany, New York.[14] A zigzag road led up the hill to the farm and was known locally as Jacob's Ladder. A pillow-shaped rock on the property prompted the place to be called Jacob's Pillow by the Carter family, the original owners.[15] It is worthy of note that the American Revolution concluded with the Treaty of Paris in 1783.

> Genesis 28 (KJV)
> 10 And Jacob went out from Beersheba, and went toward Haran.
> 11 And he lighted upon a certain place, and tarried there all
> night, because the sun was set; and he took of the stones of
> that place, and put them for his pillows, and lay down in that
> place to sleep.
> 12 And he dreamed, and behold a ladder set up on the earth,
> and the top of it reached to heaven: and behold the angels of
> God ascending and descending on it.
> 13 And behold, the Lord stood above it, and said, I am the Lord
> God of Abraham thy father, and the God of Isaac: the land
> whereon thou liest, to thee will I give it, and to thy seed…[16]

The farm was purchased 141 years later (1931) by modern dance pioneer Ted Shawn. Ted may have met Joseph Pilates in New York City and invited him to teach at Jacob's Pillow, where Joe gave lessons and taught classes from 1939 to 1951.[17] Two of the old films of Joe teaching at Jacob's Pillow are, however, dated 1932.[18]

Ted Shawn (21 October 1891 to 9 January 1972) created the Denishawn Company with his wife Ruth St. Denis about 1910.[19] The celebrated dance company, which had among its members Martha Graham, Charles Weidman, Doris Humphrey, and Jack Cole, concluded about 1929. Shawn went on to form an all-male dance company called Ted Shawn and His Men Dancers, which gave their premier performance at Jacob's Pillow in 1933. Barton Mumaw, who appears in various old photos of the 939 Studio, was a member of this dance company. Nevertheless, the films made of Joseph Pilates teaching at Jacob's Pillow show the ratio of women to men to be about 10 to 1.[20]

Joseph Pilates had still photographs of himself performing his exercises on the mat and the apparatus hung all about the 939 Studio. He also made many films, in black and white with no soundtrack, of himself and his clients performing the exercises. These films feature both men and women. Perhaps Joe meant to demonstrate that his exercises were for everyone.

It was Joe's great desire to establish his work and get it out to the world. "My work will be established and when it is, I will be the happiest man in God's Universe. My goal will have been reached."[21] It is apparent that Joe wanted everyone to practice Contrology, and that he did not care whether they were male or female. As to the dearth of men and profusion of women practitioners, perhaps this indicates that women are smarter than men! But we cannot ignore the fact that Body Contrology was created by a man, for men. I leave you to draw your own conclusions.

About Richard:

Richard Rossiter 2nd Generation Master Instructor: Richard became a Pilates instructor in 1985 and founded The Pilates Institute of Boulder, Inc. in 2000, a school for Pilates teachers, licensed by the Colorado Department of Higher Education and the Veterans Administration. Cofounded The Pilates Institute of North America, Inc., a not for profit 501(c)(3) organization that is dedicated to the rehabilitation and education of U.S. military veterans, in 2011.

REFERENCES:

1 Troy, Gordon E. R., PC, Case: Pretrial Report and Introduction. Pilates Inc. v Current Concepts, United States District Court, Southern District of New York, 96 Civ. 0043 (MGC), June 29, 2001.
2 Gallagher, Sean P. and Kryzanowska, Romana, editors. The Joseph H. Pilates Archive Collection, Photographs, Writings and Design, Bain Bridge Books, Philadelphia, PA, 2000.
3 https://en.wikipedia.org/wiki/Madison_Square_Garden
4 Grant, Kathleen Stanford: 2001 to 2010.
5 Bowen, Mary: 2001 to 2015.
6 Troy, Gordon E. R., PC, Case: Opinion, Pilates Inc. v Current Concepts, United States District Court, Southern District of New York, 96 Civ. 0043 (MGC), 2001.
7 Troy, Gordon E. R., PC, Case: Pretrial Report and Introduction. Pilates Inc. v Current Concepts, United States District Court, Southern District of New York, 96 Civ. 0043 (MGC), June 29, 2001.
8 Grimes, Jay: workshops 2009 to 2016
9 Pilates Method Alliance Conference, spring 2001. Lecture notes from presentations by Kathleen Grant, Mary Bowen, Ron Fletcher, and Lolita San Miguel.
10 http://www.pbs.org/wnet/americanmasters/tanaquil-le-clercq-about-the-film/3023/
11 Kryzanowska, Romana: Drago's Gym, 1997 to 2001.
12 Troy, Gordon E. R., PC, Case: Pretrial Report and Introduction. Pilates Inc. v Current Concepts, United States District Court, Southern District of New York, 96 Civ. 0043 (MGC), June 29, 2001.
13 Gallagher, Sean P. and Kryzanowska, Romana, editors. The Joseph H. Pilates Archive Collection, Photographs, Writings and Design, Bain Bridge Books, Philadelphia, PA, 2000.
14,15http://www.google.com/search?q=jacob's+pillow+and+Joseph+Pilates&client=safari&rls=en&gbv=2&prmd=ivns&tbm=isch&tbo=u&source=univ&sa=X&ved=0ahUKEwiwhsXH45bKAhVM5
16 Holy Bible, authorized King James Version, Collins Publishers.
17 https://en.wikipedia.org/wiki/Ted_Shawn
18 Pilates, Joseph H., Joseph H. Pilates Historic Video. These films, created by Joseph Pilates, were given to Evelyn de la Tour, who later bequeathed them to Mary Bowen. The films were then compiled and edited by Bowen who released them as a videocassette, and later as a DVD.
19 https://en.wikipedia.org/wiki/Ted_Shawn
20 Pilates, Joseph H., Joseph H. Pilates Historic Video. These films, created by Joseph Pilates, were given to Evelyn de la Tour, who later bequeathed them to Mary Bowen. The films were then compiled and edited by Bowen who released them as a videocassette, and later as a DVD.
21 Pilates, Joseph H., with Miller, William John, Your Health, 1934. (Presentation Dynamics Inc., 774 Mays Blvd, Suite 10, Incline Village, NV), 1998, 55.

Chapter V

Different Bodies, Different Minds, Positive Results

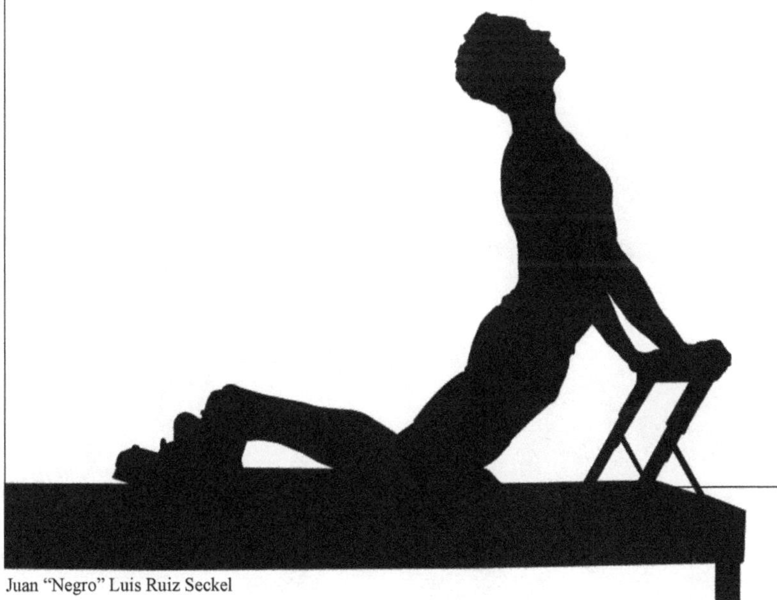

Juan "Negro" Luis Ruiz Seckel

Pilates: A Gift from My Brother

By Juan Gabriel Ruiz
Translated by Marta Cristina Diaz Velasco

> ***...once they grasp the depth of The Work, the miracle happens.***

I didn't find Pilates. It found me! At the time, I was living in the U.S., but I longed to return to my hometown, Santiago de Chile. My brother, Juan Pablo Ruiz, who owns a Pilates studio there, suggested I study the Classical Pilates system and train to become a teacher. Intrigued, I took him up on his offer to learn The Work directly from him and his wife, Veronica Zabala. But Juan Pablo made it clear that it wouldn't be easy: "You must first be a student; you must take time to understand how Pilates works in your body; you must experience the work enough to gain more self-knowledge. Then you can be sure this is really what you want." So for a year and a half, I studied, trained, performed administrative duties, and took classes, finally applying for admission to their apprenticeship program. But there was one major condition: I could only be an observer at the seminars, not an active participant, because I needed more time to explore Joe Pilates' system of mental and physical conditioning.

At the time, I experienced considerable lumbar pain, unable to remain in a standing position for more than 15 minutes. As an apprentice, though, my low back pain began to dissipate. Not long after I completed several teacher training seminars, Juan Pablo and Veronica hosted a workshop in Santiago with Peter Fiasca. His teaching truly inspired me. After attending his seminar, the Pilates system made more sense and I became even more passionate about learning and practicing The Work. I knew I had to teach Pilates!

As I began to understand The Work more deeply, and train in The Method more intelligently, I never again experienced lumbar pain. My body changed so much! As my technique improved, I became stronger, more flexible, more agile, and more coordinated than when I participated in baseball, football, and martial arts in my youth. Pilates provided me with important benefits for my daily life: good posture, energy, and muscular elongation. In a sense, it gave me back my life. On weekends, I love working with my hands in the earth, planting tomatoes, harvesting my vegetable garden, and picking fruit in the orchard. Before Pilates, I couldn't kneel in the rich soil because of back pain; now I am able to enjoy bending my knees deeply, hinging my torso forward, and reaching with my arms to work in my garden.

While I would like to say this new-found strength and flexibility resulted solely from my dedication as an apprentice, I would just be lying. It is true that I was more disciplined, I practiced and worked more hours in the studio, and I gained more technical proficiency than the other apprentices. Even though we all began at the same level, my investment paid off, and I advanced quickly. But let's give credit where credit is due; men simply have more physical strength compared to women. When you're progressing from intermediate to advanced levels, men often do so more quickly. As the only male apprentice, it was certainly easier for me to achieve the advanced level because of sheer strength. Of course, there are many exceptions; but men tend to have more physical strength, and women tend to have more physical flexibility.

But this physical strength can sometimes make it difficult for a man to grasp the depth of The Work. I have a male client who is 1.98 meters (6' feet 5" inches), 120 kilograms (264 pounds). He is tall but not fat, strong with a lot of muscle mass. Like most men, his movement comes from his arms and legs instead of from the Powerhouse; the strength originates in the periphery, and it is necessarily forced. Why? Because primary muscle groups that control arms or legs are, by definition, weaker compared to all the Powerhouse muscles, which support and distribute muscular effort through the arms or legs. Usually men force too much energy into the limbs to accomplish physical action because they are unaware of how to connect the Powerhouse with the muscles of the upper and lower extremities. Therefore "Pilates strength" can be extremely beneficial for men. In light of this fact, it's often necessary to slow men's movement so they can understand how to optimize their effort. This way, they discover Powerhouse work and properly direct strength to achieve correct action. Remember that Joe Pilates characterized Contrology as "corrective exercise." I believe this is what he meant. At the same time, however, it's important to challenge men to liberate their strength and move with coordination and dynamics because all sports involve these two skills.

Teaching Pilates to men can be challenging in other ways. From birth, men and women are socialized differently, and it is important to consider these cultural differences. Most of my clients are men. Frequently these men are managers or directors, or they have positions of responsibility; they are in charge, advising or mentoring several or many subordinates. They are not used to receiving instruction from anyone. So it's useful to give corrections in a way that doesn't make them feel like they are following orders. People have different sensibilities. As a professional Pilates teacher, you want to inspire clients, pique their interest, and help create intrigue, not occasion resistance. Although there are always exceptions, it's useful to be intuitive and diplomatic with men. Using intuition and diplomacy is essential with women, too, although they tend not to react with resistance when receiving clear instructions. I even employ different language with men as compared to women.

But once you communicate effectively with men, once they grasp the depth of The Work, the miracle happens. And they see relatively quick physical results. I have a student who is a professional race car driver. This sport is extremely demanding on the body. He suffered from severe lumbar pain and arm muscle cramps due to the intense physical work of holding and turning the steering wheel at high speeds. After a few months of Pilates training, he reported significant improvement in his lumbar discomfort and a decrease in arm muscle cramps. No more pain; no more symptoms. So very quickly!

What motivates men to study Pilates? They often start Pilates because they have an injury; they want to heal in order to resume playing their chosen sport. Others are no longer happy with their sedentary lives; they lack adequate strength and flexibility to accomplish necessary daily movements, unable to tie their shoelaces, lift a heavy suitcase, or plant a vegetable garden with relative muscular ease. In contrast, only a small percentage of women start Pilates because of an injury. Men gravitate toward The Method for very practical reasons: increasing functionality, conditioning, and stamina. They are often more focused on working hard. When I give a lesson to a man, he's present in that moment, so to speak. If I repeat a particular exercise a few times, a man will remember and know how to accomplish the exercise. They often remember how to execute movements more readily and with more confidence than women; men know how to move and where to move. In contrast, most women begin Pilates to enhance their body aesthetics, to improve posture, to lengthen and tone muscles. After a while they become interested in other aspects of the system. Yet women's initial interest in Pilates differs from the initial interest of men. Again, there are exceptions; some women remember an exercise with precision equal to a man, and some women work out with confidence similar to a man.

With all my male students, I have the same mental attitude and the same teaching approach, yet I simultaneously address the individual and his body. I always guide men in the proper ways so they can develop control and coordination, channeling their strength through movement. The Pilates system is brilliant because I can teach symptom-free men and paraplegic men with the same principles. If a student needs assistance gaining any kind of strength—physical or mental—it's part of my work to help him achieve his goal.

But not many men gravitate toward Pilates. When I reflect upon the exceptional Classical Pilates education I received under Juan Pablo and Veronica, it's unfortunate that I was the only man enrolled in their training program; all the other apprentices were women. Why is this? Why don't more men study and train to become Pilates educators? Our apprenticeship group was not unusual. Few men enter the profession. And Pilates is not popular among men here in Chile.

And marketing Pilates to men is tricky. They still perceive The Work as feminine, geared toward women. Men are less likely to participate in group classes, as they are generally populated by females. Certainly, in the beginning, it is important for novices, particularly men, to take one-on-one lessons; but Pilates is a business and no studio can survive financially by teaching private lessons. Although these students can eventually progress to Mat workouts with Wall Units and a limit of 5-6 students, again the issue of female-dominated classes arises. For a studio to be financially self-sufficient, however, Mat classes and multiple-student lessons (duets, trios, or more) as well as development of a teacher training program must be considered. I'm passionate about preserving and promoting Authentic Pilates. Yet, it's challenging to preserve Joe Pilates' traditional work and make it financially viable. But as teachers, we must persevere. We understand the importance of the work, the way it changes lives, the way it restores health. As Joseph Pilates admonished us, "Physical fitness can neither be acquired by wishful thinking nor by outright purchase. However, it can be gained through performing the daily exercises conceived for this purpose by the founder of contrology."

About Juan:

Juan Gabriel has been studying, training and teaching Joe Pilates' traditional system of corrective exercise for decades. He has developed extensive knowledge and technique throughout the years from many Classical Pilates professionals that include Dorothee VandeWalle, Kathi Ross-Nash, Jerome Weinberg, Juan Pablo Ruiz, Veronica I. Zabala and Peter Fiasca. Juan Gabriel is a physiotherapist specializing in the Pilates Method, creator of the R.R.T.P modality (rehabilitation and recovery through Pilates technology), and coordinator of the team Pilates-studio control and art.

Finding Balance

By Kyle Leith

...it remains a method that should be attractive to a much larger audience.

Pilates has been part of my life since I was nine years old. It began as an "off-ice" conditioning program to improve my figure skating, but the impact was immediate and profound. My athletic performance improved significantly as I increased my core strength, coordination, and general awareness, areas frequently lacking in young athletes. Although Pilates is rarely taught to children, I was the fortunate exception. Today, some 18 years later, although I no longer skate regularly, I still practice and now teach The Method.

My passion for Pilates led me to become one of the youngest apprentices certified by Romana's Pilates and the youngest male instructor at the time. All the male instructors I know in the industry have a tremendous passion for The Work and almost all them were greatly impacted, benefited, or even saved in some way by Pilates. While many teachers of both sexes share this passion, a male instructor in the industry will never become a teacher without it. Although rarely discussed, it's well known among men that the Pilates industry can be very unfriendly if not outright hostile to male clients and instructors. After years of teaching, I have plenty of horror stories related to the current culture of many Pilates studios. But I believe in The Work and I know that what I do helps people live better lives.

And I do retain a sense of reserved optimism when I discover studios with successful male teachers and even a surprisingly solid number of male clients. Sadly, these wonderful success stories are greatly outnumbered by the vast majority of studios with no male teachers, and no male clients. This gender imbalance caused by the poor treatment of men and a complete disregard for the male community is a growing problem. It hurts studios everywhere when the actions of a large portion of the community effectively cut the number of potential clients in half. Pilates offers men amazing and undeniable health benefits. So why is 95% of the clientele female? The answer is simple: the gradual feminization of almost every aspect of the Pilates Method.

By feminization, I mean that it has deviated from a form of exercise originally perceived as culturally masculine by the public. The Work was done primarily by males who saw the Pilates Method as something that featured elements of gymnastics and calisthenics, perceived by society at the time as masculine forms of conditioning. The feminization process occurred as a result of changes in physical movement, teaching, perception, and other qualities stereotypically linked to the female gender.

These major issues of feminization can be broken down into three categories: culture, marketing, and teaching, all of which discourage male involvement in Pilates. These factors are interconnected, intensifying over time. Current female-targeted marketing reinforces feminine Pilates stereotypes, attracting a specific type of clientele. These clients further reinforce this culture, as the needs and desires of this narrow clientele base further alter the teaching of the Pilates Method itself. By exploring, explaining, and correcting the common mistakes so many studios make regarding male clients and teachers, we can reverse the damage dealt to the male perception of Pilates and allow studios to more effectively recruit male teachers and clients.

It's often said that, "Pilates was invented by a man for men." But if you told this to the average male he would find it very difficult to believe. Joe opened up his original studio in Manhattan near the famous Madison Square Garden in hopes of training boxers. So it was a bit of a surprise when over the next several decades there was a complete gender reversal at his studio. It quickly became the training ground for a large number of high-level dancers; thus began the slow and subtle process of the feminization of the original method. Joe was well aware of the gender imbalance and was said to be disappointed because it created the public view that his method, which was intended for the human body, instead constituted physical activity for women. The Pilates Method originated with gymnastic concepts such as vigor, energy, and dynamic movement that remain an effective marketing device for stereotypically male workouts; but the perception and actual teaching of today is more focused on graceful strength and gentle, refined movement that has little appeal to the average male.

Without doubt the biggest problem preventing Pilates from attracting male clients and creating more male instructors is the Pilates culture. Defined as, "The sum of attitudes, customs, and beliefs that distinguishes one group of people from another," for our purposes, it refers to a wide range of groups, as small as a singular studio or as large as an entire certification program. Every studio is different, but many studios share similarities. One of the key shifts is the setting in which Pilates is performed. Contrology is a strenuous form of exercise, and Joe Pilates' original studio reflected that, resembling an actual gym designed for actual exercise. Today, most studios resemble something closer to a spa than a gym. I remember my first day working for a certification studio; I would never have known it was a place for exercise if it weren't for the equipment. The studio was pristine and well-kept, but I struggled to get past the smooth jazz playing faintly in the background, the Lululemon boutique, and the mood lighting. My bewilderment turned to shock when the boss told me that the studio's goal was to create a luxurious, spa-like atmosphere that made clients feel pampered. Unfortunately, many studios share this belief, but this warped concept of Pilates is so damaging that they will never succeed in having a well-rounded client base.

Pilates isn't physical therapy. Pilates isn't a dance. Pilates isn't performance art. It is a workout: a series of exercises that together create an incredible system of body conditioning that strengthens and stretches the body safely and effectively. When it isn't presented as a challenging form of exercise, then it immediately loses its appeal to men. Exercising in a "spa-like environment" is a foreign and intimidating concept to men, preventing them from ever walking in the door or taking The Method seriously. It's also not surprising that studios with similar environments tend to teach Pilates incredibly slowly, treating The Method like physical therapy or perhaps just therapy (which has value but is not Pilates). If studios want to bring in male clients, they don't have to tear down walls and suddenly look like garage gyms. They just have to remove ambient music, install normal lighting, and present the area as a place that is meant for hard work.

The studio environment is only one aspect of this changing Pilates culture. Most studios are female-dominated, making it awkward for even the most self-confident male to walk in the front door. Of the last five studios I worked at, every single employee was female. The client base of these studios was also almost entirely female, so any male client would most likely be surrounded by all women. There is nothing inherently wrong with this, but from a psychological perspective, it is intimidating, making any male feel out of place. I grew up in a female-dominated culture of figure skating, so I have never really been impacted by disproportionate male/female ratios; however, the issue becomes very clear when I try to convince male friends/family to give Pilates a try. This could be remedied by marketing to men or hiring male instructors who could further the concept that Pilates isn't just for women.

I wish I could say that my complaints about the current culture of Pilates ended with simplistic comments on atmosphere, but, unfortunately, my considerable experience in the Pilates community has led me to conclude that male clients are often unwelcome and generally treated differently. While ostensibly male teachers are beloved, in reality they face a great deal of sexism and double standards absent elsewhere in the fitness industry. This is where passion becomes a necessity. If it weren't for resiliency and a love of teaching, I'd have quit a hundred times over. During my Pilates certification, I was the only male apprentice among women. Over the next five months of training, I was forced to practice and train alone much of the time. Since I struggled to find apprentices willing to work with a male, I had to practice teach my girlfriend and whatever friends she could recruit as practice bodies. While this was a hardship, it was the key to my early success as a teacher. It's easy to teach an apprentice who knows exactly what he is doing, but the real learning process for an instructor begins the first time he works with a client who knows nothing and tries to lie down on the Reformer backwards.

My difficulties adjusting to the female-centric culture of Pilates continued as a certified teacher, facing the harsh reality that wherever I worked nearly a quarter of the clients wouldn't train with me simply because I was male. None of them had met me, seen me teach, or heard a bad word about me, but they refused to study with me because of my gender. This became painfully evident when I substituted for a chronically ill instructor whose clients were used to having subs; over the course of five hours, three clients walked in the door and promptly declared, “No offense, but I don’t work with male instructors.” After demanding refunds, they left. This is an all too common experience for most male teachers, but it is one that has become widely accepted with a simple shoulder shrug by the Pilates community. Clearly, this is a learned response; during the three years I worked as a personal trainer, I never once had a client refuse to work with me because I was male.

If these experiences weren’t enough to discourage me from my career path, I soon faced an even more uncomfortable situation. The owner of a large studio at which I had just been hired asked if I were homosexual. When I introduced my girlfriend, who was nearby looking at the boutique, the owner looked disappointed. Without batting an eye, she inquired, “May I tell clients that you are anyway? It might drum up business?” My girlfriend laughed, but I was offended by the suggestion, politely replying, “I’d rather not say and just let my teaching speak for itself.” She nodded and agreed. But the following day, in an email blast to the clientele, she introduced me, posting a picture of me with my girlfriend (who had unknowingly had her picture taken). Furthermore, my boss decided I was now married, too, as that would make me less threatening to female clients. It’s this culture and negative perception of male teachers that makes it difficult to hire new instructors, compounded by second class status, low salary, no benefits, and zero safety net. I’ve seen very little that would lead me to believe there is change coming for Pilates instructors outside of having studio owners who are brave enough to hire male teachers and not use them as puppets to convince female clients to buy a couples package and bring their husbands to work out.

Another factor hurting male participation in Pilates is marketing. I could write a book as long as *War and Peace* about how poorly marketed Pilates is in regard to recruiting men. But even the most egregious errors can be avoided. Currently, if most Pilates studios did absolutely zero advertising of any kind, they would position themselves better than they currently are when it comes to recruiting male clients. Most studios don’t advertise to men, but even worse, they market to females so strongly that it indirectly pushes male clients away.

When I was first introduced to Pilates, I was far too young to have even the slightest idea of what The Method was, let alone the public perception of it. My skating coach, Karen Courtland Kelly, told me that Pilates would help my skating, and that was the end of the conversation. Unfortunately, most people don't have the good fortune to receive a convincing sales pitch on the benefits of Pilates from a former Olympic athlete. In hindsight, if it weren't for the guidance of Karen, for whom I have the utmost respect, I would never have considered participating in Pilates as an adult. My male ego and natural levels of self-consciousness would have ruled it out based on the modern presentation of Pilates in infomercials, magazine articles, newsletters, and Internet posts. It's hard to express how negative the male view of The Method is. Suffice it to say that most female Pilates instructors have Facebook profiles of themselves doing Teasers or other Pilates exercises. Many male instructors don't even tell their own friends that they teach Pilates, let alone post pictures of themselves doing Pilates exercises.

What could be so appalling about Pilates marketing that it alienates the majority of men? Perception. Most men perceive Pilates as floor exercises for "dainty" women who are afraid to lift weights, and the system itself is often categorized as a fad similar to jazzercise and aerobics. These stereotypes were well, deserved and reinforced over the course of many years through extremely effective marketing in the early 1990s. The campaigns used infomercials to introduce The Method to the public as a mat workout for women who wanted to tone and slim down. The damage from these ad campaigns launched 20 years ago can still be felt today as men continue to perceive The Work as a series of floor exercises featuring middle-aged women squeezing magic circles for 45 minutes straight. While this is the furthest thing from the truth, it doesn't matter because in business, perception is reality. In a recent article in *Men's Fitness*, a writer found out his assignment was to attend a Pilates class; from the overly sexualized covers he frequently saw featured on *Pilates Monthly*, he envisioned Pilates as a brand of "ballerina yoga." Obviously, his assumptions were wrong, but it is this damaging perception that has prevented Pilates from reaching the levels of success that it should garner.

I'd like to think the mistakes in marketing end with infomercials, but many studios buy into the idea that "Pilates is for women." This notion just intensifies the client gender imbalance, alienating potential male clients. Reversing the trend requires a change in advertising.

Common marketing mishaps are often obvious, but somehow infinitely repeated:

1) Not marketing to men. If a studio doesn't make an effort to bring in male clients, they won't. The biggest mistake is not even trying to attract men to Pilates, and this is by far the most common mistake in modern marketing. It doesn't require specific ads directed at men but small changes like a picture of a male client on a Reformer could go a very long way.

2) Not hiring male teachers. Many studios claim that they would love to have a male instructor, but that is rarely the case. It's extremely difficult to be a male teacher in most Pilates studios today, but hiring one brings tremendous credibility to the studio when it comes to attracting male clients.

3) Newsletter blasts targeting women only. When I worked for a studio in Saratoga, I received at least 20 emails about classes to get in "bikini shape" or workshops to strengthen the "pelvic floor." I'd be hard pressed to find a way to alienate men quicker.

4) Sexualized marketing often featured in the likes of *Pilates Style*. Marketing Pilates sox on an otherwise nude model furthers false perceptions about Pilates, alienating male (and probably many female) clients.

The last crucial element that has been feminized over time is the actual Pilates Method and how it's taught, particularly in the past ten years. Joe preached vigor, flow, and strong movements. I am not referring to the dangerously fast pace of derivative styles of Pilates; that is not the classical work. Joe just emphasized movement more than the way someone held his hands in an exercise. Today the dynamic rhythm and pacing, hallmarks of the traditional system, have been replaced by a focus on over correction and excessive tactile cuing. The pace of teaching in many classical studios has slowed to a crawl. This is the result of several generations of former dancers training dancers, losing sight of the male workmanlike quality Joe taught his clients or the energy for which Romana was famous. Dancer culture has made

The Work incredibly detail, orientated, appearing out of tune with men and modern fitness. Even the cuing alienates male clients. Telling a man to "pull down your wings" elicits either a cringe or an eye roll. And what man wants to hear a teacher say, "Isn't this delicious?" (This is a common Pilates saying that originated from an extremely sexualized scene by Marilyn Monroe.)

The biggest disappointment is that almost all the masculine calisthenic movements have been removed from the system, and many of the more masculine and strength, related exercises such as pushups are rarely taught. I find it depressing that in today's Pilates system, most certifications require teachers to know countless variations of the "Splits," but few know any of the advanced Arm Springs, which are considered archival. The results, however, speak for themselves when the majority of Pilates instructors can't do more than five push-ups!

Pilates should be extremely easy to sell to men. The use of springs mimics popular methods of resistance training and the use of straps on the Reformer and Cadillac share many similarities with the TRX exercise system that is currently in fashion. When Pilates is taught with solid flow and well-performed transitions, it can be cardiovascular, similar to HIIT (High Intensity Interval Training), which is without question one of the most popular forms of exercise for men and athletes of all kinds throughout the world today. The key point is that Pilates is still ahead of its time almost 50 years after Joe's death. When taught correctly, it remains a method that should be attractive to a much larger audience. But if the level of teaching is diminished, improved culture and marketing are irrelevant.

Pilates is often called a lifetime journey, and while this sounds clichéd, it's true. As an instructor, I have realized that I learn something new almost every day. However, like many others, I tend to forget something every day as well—sometimes a minor detail, or a cue, or a random piece of information. It's common to forget what we don't teach, and for me that's super advanced work, but for many others it's how to teach male clients. The most common error in teaching male clients is inappropriate spotting. Never stand in front of a client during Pelvic Lift. Always teach with cupped hands similar to a swimmer. It's important to spot, but it's equally important to realize that most clients are not dancers, and they don't have the same comfort level as an athlete who has been poked and prodded by coaches and trainers. In short, awareness is everything. Everybody is different, and it's always better to be safe than sorry.

The goal of every Pilates instructor should be to provide the client with a safe, effective, and enjoyable workout. If the teacher fails at any of these three things, either the client will not come back, or he will not get results.

Consider the following:

1A) Safety (physical): Obviously, this is the most important factor. If a client is injured, he doesn't get results, he is unhappy, and in the majority of cases he sues the instructor.
1B) Safety (emotional): This element of the workout is frequently overlooked. It's about feeling safe with the instructor. If the client doesn't trust the teacher or feel at ease with him then there is a problem. Pilates is full of unflattering, awkward positions. If the teacher can't remain completely professional at all times or can't make the client feel safe and comfortable, he will not come back.

2) Effectiveness: If Pilates doesn't produce results, then it's time to reevaluate your teaching. It is a powerful method that changes every body. If all your clients look and feel the same as they did six months ago, YOU will notice. And, trust me when I say, they will notice, too. Nobody in his right mind spends hundreds of dollars for a workout that fails to produce results.

3) Fun: This is the most important point. Most clients will tell you that Pilates is HARD, but they LOVE it. They go to class every week with smiles on their faces, and they leave happy and invigorated. That is what all Pilates instructors, strive for, because if your client is having fun, he is more likely to come back. The word fun is rarely attributed to exercise, but perhaps that is why so many people in this country don't work out! Fun can mean many things, but to a Pilates instructor it generally translates to: "I feel great after my workout. At no point was I ever bored, and I definitely want to come back."

If the goal of a Pilates session is a safe, effective, and fun workout, it's amazing how many teachers fail to complete all three. Failure to achieve the first objective, safety, is generally due to poor training or substandard certification. Overworked teachers suffering from burn-out can also fall short of the mark. Once client safety is compromised, the workout cannot be effective or fun. It is a domino effect.

The critical error is losing balance. Not actual physical balance, but teaching balance—finding the thin line between teaching proper form and allowing the student to move uncorrected. Having a proper balance between these two extremes is the key to being effective as a teacher. Although the two teaching styles are polar opposites of each other, both destroy the essence of Classical Pilates espoused by its creator.

The "movement" teacher focuses on physical activity and rarely makes corrections. Going from one exercise to the next with great speed and little attention to form, this instructor can cover countless exercises in a short period of time, often tricking people into thinking Pilates is a spin class taught on the ground. This style of teaching can be effective, but it is generally dangerous. Minimal correction leads to bad form, bad habits, and bad backs. Pilates believes in quality over quantity; a few good repetitions of an exercise are better than many executed badly.

The "form" teacher is all about creating the perfect shape. He teaches slowly, very slowly. Everything is calculated, aligned, and symmetrical. This teacher talks constantly about the "Powerhouse" and uses touch excessively. In one hour, the client barely completes mat work, which normally takes 20-25 minutes at a respectable pace. Until the form is perfect, the student cannot go on to the next exercise. This style of teaching can be good if you're working with an injured client or a professional dancer who needs to have considerable body control. Teaching good form also tends to be safer; the client learns the form over time, and eventually is able to work at a faster pace. But the average client who isn't used to being so heavily corrected and analyzed often leaves the lesson feeling discouraged. Generally, teaching at such a slow pace destroys a workout, but some teachers can get away with it; they still have clients dripping wet from sweat. These teachers are few and far between.

The two extremes both have some benefits, but they fail miserably to achieve the goals of Pilates. Finding the balance between these two opposite styles is crucial in maintaining and building a clientele. But this is not an easy task! I have taught a while, and sometimes I have a tendency to move a little too fast or go a little too slow. If a teacher professes to always teach at a proper pace, then he is lying, or just resistant to self-examination and self-improvement.

Here are some quick tips on how to become a balanced teacher:

1) Corrections: Every correction should make the exercise safer, more effective, or, in general, more correct. In other words, if your correction isn't about safety, improving, or enhancing the workout, then it's not worth making. Having someone's hands look "pretty" is not worth stopping a person who is paying $1.25 a minute.

2) Talking: Be aware of it. Try to stay on topic if possible, and try to make the client focus on the exercise at hand. DON'T talk to prevent silence. Some of the best lessons I have ever had didn't involve much talking at all. There is already enough for the client to think about!

3) Touch: Don't touch your client on every exercise. The best advice I ever received was that when you touch a client, it better be meaningful. Never "half" spot somebody. If you make a correction, MAKE THE CORRECTION. Otherwise, you are just in the way.

4) Efficiency: The fastest way to speed up a workout is transitions. This is the time between exercises. If you are slow to adjust the reformer or get the client into the next position, then you can easily waste 10 minutes or $15 of your client's time. They may not notice at first, but if they work with a teacher who does transitions quickly they will notice. That reflects poorly on you.

5) Good decisions: Not everything has to be perfect or correct. As a teacher, you pick your battles. The human mind can only remember about three corrections at a time. So why overload it and then hope that the client remembers the important corrections? A good instructor should have a focus during the lesson. Maybe that means being strict with Stomach Massage and less picky on Knee Stretches, for example. A good teacher applies these principles to every body, male or female.

And a good teacher welcomes working with a diverse clientele. But the industry isn't where it needs to be if it wants to increase the number of male clients and teachers in the future. This is due to poor marketing, an unwelcoming culture for men, and teaching that has replaced the masculine exercises with a focus on elements that are unappealing to men. Thankfully there are still many great teachers out there who welcome male clients and teachers and leave me optimistic that more men will experience the same benefits that I did from Pilates.

About Kyle:

Kyle Leith has been a certified Pilates instructor since 2008 and has worked in New York City, Connecticut, Philadelphia, and Amherst, Massachusetts. He is also a certified personal trainer and has worked with high-level athletes.

Pilates: The Mind-Body Connection

By Emre Onuk

Mastering these challenging exercises really motivates men.

Turkey is not exactly the first place that comes to mind when referring to the epicenter of the Pilates world, but I am proud to belong to a small yet faithful community of Turkish men and women whose lives have been changed for the better through Pilates. My path to The Work came about through my profession, a soloist with the Ankara State Ballet. I sustained a number of knee and shoulder injuries requiring surgery, a shinbone fracture, and a hernia. My joints were practically devoid of cartilage. The doctors told me I might never walk again, and all seemed hopeless—until, that is, I discovered the power of Pilates in 2003. It is to this miraculous system I give credit for my now pain-free life and the laughs I share with my doctors when we recall their grim prophecies.

My introduction to The Work began with several neo-Pilates systems, but the actual change in my life occurred when I found Peter Fiasca's DVDs. Later, I had the great privilege of working with him for an extended period in London, after which he sent me to my dear teacher, Marjorie Oron, founder of the first European Pilates studio in the Netherlands. I will be grateful forever to these two incomparable teachers.

Through their masterful teaching and guidance, I regained my strength and healed from my injuries. But the system gave me a far greater gift, a deeply emotional and personal one; by introducing my wife, ballerina Özge Başaran Onuk, to Pilates, I helped her return to the stage after cruciate ligament surgery. Throughout my career as a Pilates instructor, I have had many students who were athletes and dancers, and conversely those who were businesspeople or led sedentary lifestyles, all of whom benefited from The Work.

Pilates is considered by many to be the realm of women, a method solely for weight control and body shaping. This is particularly true in Turkey. Unfortunately, just as in many other countries, this means that women fall prey to scams by uneducated and careless instructors and entrepreneurs unconcerned with what Pilates really entails. In the fitness market, businesses bastardize The Work, splicing it up, combining it with other disciplines, and generally distorting it beyond recognition in order to attract women as customers. This not only means that women are shortchanged but also that men are left without a chance to discover the great benefits of Pilates.

Anyone who knows about Joseph Pilates and his revolutionary approach to the human body understands that the so-called Pilates and fitness trends marketed by modern businesses have nothing to do with his character and philosophy. They have everything to do with greed. My team and I struggle against these inaccurate perceptions of Pilates and, fortunately, have become the first in our field in Turkey to organize a number of workshops, seminars, and conferences on authentic Classical Pilates.

Men and women who come to our events are often surprised to find out that Pilates is much more than a fad designed for superficial female beautification. As we teach in our exercise classes, workshops and conferences, the logic behind the Pilates system is the control of mind over body, resulting in perfect harmony of body and mind. Pilates cannot be confined within the narrow boundaries of an exercise system: while our students do report better weight control, greater core strength, and improved flexibility with Pilates, they are also pleased to discover other effects that greatly contribute to their well-being.

All of our students live in large cities and are subject to the ravages of city life: their posture is deplorable, not only due to the forces of gravity exerted on a weak spine, common to all people, but exacerbated by work days spent at desks or hunched over clients. Lack of exercise is very common in Turkey, especially among men over 30, and a diet based mainly on carbohydrates is the norm. Most, if not all, experience stress which, together with a sedentary lifestyle, bad diet and poor posture, leads to a host of emotional issues and psychosomatic ailments, as well as stiffness, constant fatigue, tension, and muscle aches.

Those who are, in their own words, lucky enough to discover Pilates have found that this system is more than just a way to burn calories; most of our male students are surprised to discover that muscles are stretched as much as they are exercised, providing energy and well-being. The torso and hips are less flexible in males than in females, especially when deprived of exercise and distorted into unhealthy posture. Pilates provides significant relief by stretching these areas and making them suppler, thus counteracting stress and tension. Furthermore, the improvement in muscle strength and flexibility is so rewarding for men that it fuels even greater progress.

Men respond to Pilates differently from women. The fact that it was developed by a man, for men, probably explains why I am able to teach my male students more easily and communicate with them more efficiently in the studio. While women often have a hard time with demanding exercises like pushups and handstands, men prefer these exercises precisely because they are challenging. Our male students love the Powerhouse series and exercises like swakate, rowing series, arm springs, and kneeling arm circles. They enjoy feeling the bulk of the weights against their arms. Mastering these challenging exercises really motivates men, probably due to the release of dopamine; in turn, this feeling of success or accomplishment promotes consistency and commitment to the exercise regimen and leads to a general feeling of well-being in all areas of life.

The emotional and psychological impact of Pilates appears to be the most important benefit for our students; they uniformly report that Pilates develops more than just their muscles. This is especially true for men. What distinguishes Pilates from other systems is that it develops the body symmetrically, providing the exercises each individual body needs, while improving emotional health and cognitive capability. The starting point of Pilates, after all, is the control of the mind over the muscles; and since mind and body are part of the same indivisible organism, as the exercise is continued with persistence and discipline, inevitably the mind will improve just as the muscles do.

One form that this takes is improved concentration. As the mind is disciplined together with the body, and taught to focus on the task at hand, the muscles are focused on mastering a certain exercise. The other related consequence is that the feelings of well-being, motivation and satisfaction overcome the fatigue, depression, and lack of confidence that are so often an integral part of modern life.

Depression is no less real here than in Western countries. Most often, this is especially a problem for men, because admitting feelings of defeat or acknowledging a mental health issue is seen as weak and unmanly. While women can discuss emotional issues with friends or tackle these problems with self-help books, often the only so-called solutions for men are alcohol and violent altercations, which just exacerbate their problems.

To those men weighed down not only by their guts, but also by stress, fatigue, and feelings of inadequacy and loneliness, Pilates has brought invaluable relief. What makes their lives better is not only the gain in muscle mass and flexibility, but improved motivation, self-confidence, and the trust in the increased capacity of the mind and body. In our courses and events, we have witnessed this time and time again.

Recently, a CEO reluctantly started Pilates after realizing that his lifestyle up to that point had done nothing to alleviate his problems. He did not have a sedentary lifestyle by any means: he swam, jogged, and lifted weights. But apart from that, he was a textbook example of the overworked, overstressed successful businessman. Frequent business trips and long meetings meant a disturbed circadian rhythm and, more often than not, poor diet. He was stressed and prone to anger. Despite a rigorous exercise regimen, he had the stiffest body I have ever seen. Wealthy as he was, the poor fellow could not bend to pick up a coin from the ground. His back and neck were practically wooden, and muscle pain and lack of energy made his life a living hell.

Before long, the system he initially described as "some girly thing he'd been talked into," transformed this rigid ball of pain into an energetic, strong man who can kick as high as he stands. His back pain has been supplanted by strong back muscles, his fatigue by boundless energy. However, he asserts that the physical improvements are nothing compared to the mental ones; he is now better able to concentrate, not only on his exercises, but also on crucial details in his work projects. This has greatly lessened his stress and made him a happier man who is generally more pleasant to be around.

Fortunately, we meet a lot of students who recover from physical ailments and injuries with the help of Pilates, like the hotel owner and passionate cyclist whose knee surgeries had not only forced him to stop cycling, but also allegedly required extensive surgery. Pilates did away with the pains in his knees, and he was able to resume cycling within months.

Other students similarly benefited from Pilates in combating spine and posture problems related to their professions: a dentist, who enjoyed competitive ballroom dancing, experienced severe back pain and was unable to maintain good posture simply because he stood hunched over his patients eight hours a day. Pilates reduced his pain, improved his performance on the dance floor, and generally improved his life so much that he is considering teaching Pilates for a living.

Another student with similar, job-related problems owns a high-end hair salon. Cutting and styling hair on his feet all day meant perpetually stiff and aching muscles from his neck and back all the way down to his legs. His social life appeared satisfying at first sight, but socializing almost every night brought with it the consumption of copious amounts of alcohol and trouble adapting to the job environment the morning after. He was not only continually tired, he was unhappy, tense and depressed.

Pilates remedied both his physical and emotional issues. The exercises cured his aches and pains, while the discipline motivated him to tackle his life and implement serious lifestyle changes. Healthier social relationships, including romantic developments, made for a better social life. Less alcohol coupled with exercise led to more energy. And the new outlook on life gained through Pilates made him both more capable and more creative at his job.

All these men had tried the common marketplace remedies for their problems: over-the-counter, prescription, or herbal drugs; expensive diet plans; fitness and sports sessions taught by inexperienced and careless instructors. It was only when they adopted the Pilates system and complemented strength with concentration that they could realize what their bodies, and their minds, were capable of. They gained flexibility and muscle mass, but more importantly, they gained confidence and courage.

None of this would have been possible with the common exercise and weight loss methods on the market. It would also not have been possible with the watered-down, distorted, commercialized Pilates that is peddled to unwitting customers. It is my hope that in Turkey, as in the world, true and valuable Pilates will be distinguished from the repackaged, corrupted versions currently flooding the market. The physical, mental, and social improvements that our students have experienced in their lives should, after all, be available to all men.

About Emre:

Emre originally started Pilates in 2002. During 2007, Emre trained intensively with Peter Fiasca in Authentic Pilates. Inspired to gain further education in Traditional Pilates, Emre then studied extensively under the supervision of world-renowned Marjorie Oron at The Pilates Studio in The Hague. At the same time, Emre trained closely with Jane Poerwoatmodjo and consolidated his knowledge with all talented instructors at the Romana's Pilates organization, including Romana Kryzanowska's daughter, Sari Mejia Santo. During 2015, Emre was promoted to Level 4 Instructor within the Romana's Pilates family of teachers. Emre is thankful and inspired to help preserve Joe Pilates' original system of mental and physical conditioning.

Pilates for Men

By Corinne Dawson

> ***Pilates is perfectly suited to bring more balance to the male body.***

Over the years, countless female clients have asked if I would teach Pilates to their husbands. I usually tell them if they can just get their husbands in the door, Pilates can work miracles for them. Many of those clients have asked me about the difference between teaching Pilates to men versus women. The truth is that on some level Pilates is the same for everyone, but since men are different from women in many ways, we cannot teach them in the exact same way. Romana loved working with men. In workshops, she always chose them to demonstrate. At first I thought it was just a fun change of pace for her, but with more experience, I learned how Pilates is perfectly suited to bring more balance to the male body. Certain elements of Classical Pilates as taught to me by Romana bring unique benefits to men. It can change the way a man moves in a very short period of time and open his eyes to a whole new approach to his body.

Women like myself, training to become Pilates instructors in the '90s, were a dime a dozen. For every 30 women enrolled in the teacher certification program, there were one or two men. As apprentices learning The Work, the gender differences were noticeable. While I could perform many advanced Pilates exercises with relative ease and precision, there were other elements of the system clearly designed by a man, for men. Exercises like the One Armed Twist, Star, and the Standing Arm Springs are clearly designed for a man's shoulders. It is breathtaking to witness the power, rhythm, and strength of Pilates when a strong, flexible man executes The Work. The lines are perfect. That is why Romana loved working with men.

When I started teaching in my late 20s, on average, I had ten female clients to every male client. I quickly learned that while you could teach the same movements to both groups, you could not teach the same way. Men and women approach The Work with completely different goals, personalities, strengths, and weaknesses. Seventeen years later, that ratio has changed, and today I have three women to every male client. I have taught several husband and wife duets, the wife dragging the husband in to see her Pilates studio, and the husband often ending up more committed to Pilates than his spouse. What a joy to work with a variety of people and to see them all hungry for that wonderful, tall, strong feeling you experience at the end of your session!

I have taken countless workshops on how to teach Pilates to male clients. They are very helpful, mostly because they are often taught by exceptional male instructors who tell their own Pilates stories. They speak from experience about the different approaches and different language that facilitate teaching men. And they teach the "men's exercises," advanced movements focusing on the upper body. It is always helpful for me to review the men's repertoire, as I rarely teach it. These exercises require so much control that it is not always possible or necessary for my male clients to execute them in order to grow and change in incredible ways. Most of my male clients are over 55, and they pursue Pilates as a means to an end. They come in to get a better golf score, to stay the same height, to feel less back pain. One client started Pilates because he was so inflexible he could no longer tie his shoe laces. The specific goal brings them in; but when the Pilates bug bites, they are hooked.

The magic in teaching Pilates is finding out what the client is missing and how to communicate that to him so he feels it in his own body. I learned a lot about teaching through intuition and trial and error. As a new teacher, it would have been helpful to read some case studies of male clients. The technical part of Pilates is easy to teach once you've figured out the personality traits of the student and the techniques to teach him effectively. Here are a few stories from inside a Pilates studio—lessons learned from my male clients...

A Lesson in Awareness:

A 50-year-old surgeon walked into the studio, demanding, "Tell me why I should do this Pilates stuff. This place looks like a torture chamber. I already stretch and do core work all the time, and it doesn't work. I am still tight, and I get cramps. This is just a bunch of hocus-pocus!"

I thought to myself, *With that attitude I should send him to a yoga studio or foist him on another trainer...* but I suggested that if he were already stretching and working hard independently with little or no results, he may need to look for a new approach to solve the problem. I cautioned him that Pilates isn't for everyone, but that over and over again, I have seen it help many people in many ways. Despite himself, he signed up for his first lesson, although he looked quite nervous when he arrived.

In the first 20 minutes of the lesson, he experienced over twenty muscle cramps. A simple bit of footwork on the Reformer or light spring work on the Cadillac sent him hobbling about the room in pain. He informed me there was no medical reason for the cramps, and his body had been like that since his youth. His father never allowed him to swim as a child, fearing he would suffer cramps and drown.

What was I going to do with him? Whenever I am stumped by a new client, I just pass along The Work of Joseph Pilates as it was conveyed to me by Romana and Juanita. I took him to the mat and explained the most basic principles of The Work: The Box, The Powerhouse, working towards more balance between stretch and strength in the body. Surprisingly, he could execute a decent Roll-up and a few good pushups. At the end of the session, I booked his next few lessons!

By his fourth session, we were down to two muscle cramps. And he began to notice structural misalignments without any prompting from me. So we focused on increasing body awareness, moving with precision, and improving body control through better concentration. He also began to smile and relax a bit. After 10 lessons he was standing up taller, moving better, and experiencing very little cramping. He also confessed to noticing that everyone in his office had terrible posture, and he had begun telling them that they all needed to do Pilates. He went from a doubting Thomas to a Pilates disciple! I recently heard him tell a client working out next to him that I must have thought he was a real jerk when he first came in, but that he was glad I took him on anyway!

I find this story amusing now, but it is also fascinating to compare his experience to that of many female clients who generally take longer to progress. Pilates, sometimes in spite of the client, works wonders for men—often in a very short amount of time. I have wondered why they progress so quickly in Pilates, and in part it is the physical activities they enjoy as children. Unlike women, most of my male clients played sports in their youth, later working out at a gym, running, or cycling. The introduction of Pilates evokes new sensations and heightened body awareness, resulting in a seismic shift in movement efficiency.

A Lesson in Persistence:

My father began taking group mat classes regularly a few years ago. That's when I discovered what a gift it is to teach someone you love; suddenly you view them from a different perspective. Instead of seeing a man who is my dad, I observed someone who had worked through innumerable injuries and medical issues with absolute grace. I also saw someone who was open to learning new skills and applying them to other areas of his life. Most of all, I saw someone who just kept showing up and doing the best he could over and over again. He was stiff and awkward in class for a long time, so I made sure he was working safely, but I pretty much left him alone to do the best he could.

One day, about a year into his training, I looked over toward his corner of the room, just as his hips floated up off the ground in a beautiful Rollover. I would not have guessed it possible, but Pilates just works if you keep at it! Finding a way to encourage clients to be consistent and give the body time to change is the challenge. Sometimes even the teacher is amazed at how well Pilates works!

A Lesson in Embracing the Gray Area:

A few years ago, a gentleman in his late 50s entered the Pilates studio, inquiring whether Pilates could help him gain flexibility. He explained that he had just finished cardiac rehab and was doing well, but his muscles were tight. I set up a lesson, and as we reviewed his health history, he confessed that as a professor of statistics, he feels most comfortable in the realm of numbers and computers. As an adult, he never really explored exercise until his doctor forced him into a cardiac rehab program at the wellness center housing the Pilates studio where I work. During his first few lessons, he appeared slightly confused and uncomfortable. At the conclusion of the third lesson, he admitted that he did not understand how I could tell if he was improving over time. How could I quantify his progress? Weight, blood pressure, and many other numbers denoted improvement in his cardiac rehab program, but how could I tell if he were doing well in Pilates?

I explained that in the Pilates system of movement, most clients begin with the Basic work; and as they progress, they learn bits of the intermediate exercises when appropriate. At some point, anywhere from several months to several years, they become strong intermediates and may even execute some advanced movements. We use our knowledge, intuition, and experience as teachers to move clients along at the correct pace. The end goal for every person, however, is not to achieve the full advanced Pilates system. The end goal is to gain more awareness, better alignment, and control year after year. Young apprentices must learn and perform every exercise they plan on teaching, but most clients have more important lessons to learn. Finally, I asked him if he feels better after his lessons. Smiling, he admitted that he felt taller and his spirits were lifted. He noted that I seemed quite comfortable in what felt like a gray area to him, intimating that further exploration of Pilates may benefit him in ways he had never imagined.

A true Pilates Evangelist, this man now tells everyone about the benefits of the work. Thanks to Pilates, he moves better and feels better. He has joined a masters' swim team, goes snowboarding, plays tennis, and even takes tap class. His cardiac issues and ensuing exploration of movement have changed his life. Now he is on a constant quest to achieve freedom of movement, strength, and flexibility, quantifiable or not!

A Lesson in Being Manly:

Once a week, I teach a mat class for students at a local university. For several semesters, one of the regular participants was a star of the men's baseball team. Young and muscular, he could easily have been a fitness model; although he was very strong in some ways, he often experienced pain in his back and hips. The right side of his body was dramatically stronger and tighter than his left. But his commitment to The Work paid off, and he improved quickly. One day he confessed that his back had hurt for several years, but after Pilates class it always felt better. When I asked if he had ever gone to the doctor or spoken with a coach about it, he laughed, explaining that guys don't show their weakness to coaches or fellow players. Telling his female Pilates teacher about his back pain felt safe. And it gave me the opportunity to help him discover ways to apply Pilates concepts to his daily life, other training regimes, and sports.

It is a shame that sometimes men hide discomfort or weakness from one another. In this case, it was a common problem with a relatively simple solution. Several of my male clients confided that they don't tell male personal trainers, Pilates instructors, or coaches when something hurts them because they don't want to complain or appear weak. That information is vital to choosing the right program for the client. Pilates is not physical therapy, but it can be therapeutic. When a man explores his weaknesses and uses Pilates to address them, his sports performance improves dramatically. Being able to create a space where the man does not feel so competitive or "manly" is a good thing.

A Lesson in Control:

For several years now, I have been teaching a gentleman who suffered such severe back pain it interrupted his sleep and prevented him from playing golf. He had heard Pilates could help him, and he thought he would give me a chance to prove it! As a CEO, he has tremendous responsibility and pressure in his life. When he spoke about work, I watched the tension increase, his body getting tighter with each sentence. At first he was nervous about his back and even more nervous about stepping into the Pilates world. He was a man used to feeling confident, in control. It took quite a while to help him become the teachable and trusting client he is today.

It is often not the body, but the personality we need to be most aware of as we teach a new client. This client often began his lesson with a negotiation. He might suggest that instead of doing the Tree that morning, we should do those Barrel Stretches. Or instead of the Teaser, we could do some extra Roll-Ups on the mat. I was as flexible as I needed to be to keep him coming back until he started to trust that Pilates works—if you work it. He began to marvel at how tired he was after doing 8 repetitions of Elephant correctly. And he moved with more freedom and body integration in his everyday life. And his golf game became more fluid. For him, the biggest lesson he learned in

Pilates is to let go of control both mentally and physically. He learned to trust that someone else could lead the way. And he learned to release the tight, overworked external muscles that were causing him discomfort, allowing the deeper muscles of The Center lead the way. Letting go of control changed him significantly.

Who Should Teach the Men?

I have talked with several fellow Pilates instructors about whether male clients benefit more from working with male or female instructors. This is a real dilemma for me. Having taught many male clients, I watched them transform the way they move, the way they think about their bodies. Instinctively, I have created a comfortable space where men can explore their weaknesses and learn to work well, and even breathe at the same time. On the occasions when these men work with male instructors, they come right back to me looking for that space where they can let their guard down, concentrate, and work hard.

On the other hand, a male Pilates instructor understands, from the inside out, what it feels like to have the shoulders and hips of a man. And it is easier to provide the perfect explanation or cue for any exercise when you have a similar body type. This parallels my understanding of what it feels like to do Pilates while pregnant. I can describe it to my male colleagues and teach them all they need to know to do it safely, but I have experienced it from the inside. That is priceless when relating to the client and making good intuitive choices while teaching them. When I have a male client who is really progressing and interested in studying Pilates on a much deeper level, or considering getting certified, I suggest they work with male and female instructors alike. I have benefited greatly from taking lessons from a variety of amazing Pilates masters. A female instructor with a body similar to mine often knows all of my tricks before they even happen. On the flip side, I have a colleague who is an amazing male Pilates instructor. He has traveled and studied with most of the best men in the Pilates world. He excels at performing an advanced exercise that has always been very difficult for me called the Star. When a male client of mine gets to that level, I have them work together on it.

It is important for our male clients to learn that Pilates is for everyone. Joseph Pilates was a man who worked with men and women. His gym did not have a spa-like atmosphere with mood music playing in the background. It is serious stuff, challenging for the mind and the body. Classical Pilates, when taught well, works wonders. Good alignment and efficient movement is not just for girls anymore!

About Corinne:

As a college student at the University of Iowa in 1992, Corinne took her first Pilates mat class. Almost instantly, her flexible body felt more connected than ever before. It seemed clear that Pilates was something she needed to explore. After dancing for several years after college, she began working with several Pilates instructors in Chicago, learning more about The Method and the certifications available. Soon she found Juanita Lopez, who taught her almost everything she knows about Pilates. Juanita is one of the ultimate authorities in the world on Classical Pilates. Romana, Sari, and other Master teachers came from New York for weeks, teaching, leading seminars, and testing apprentices. In 1998, Corinne began teaching clients at Pilates studios, fitness clubs, and dance studios in Chicago. She helped build a thriving studio in a hospital wellness center, and she currently owns a studio in the Northern suburbs of Chicago.

Muscle Balance and Longevity Through Pilates

By Alessandro Balboni

...absolutely applicable to all males to help them become stronger, achieve greater performance...

Vitality and strength are immediately reflected in the way we feel and appear. Joe Pilates wrote, "Contrology is designed to give you suppleness, natural grace, and skill that will be unmistakably reflected in the way you walk, in the way you play, and in the way you work."

I am 47 years old. Throughout my life I have devoted myself to physical conditioning and sports. Some disciplines are very strenuous. I have demanded peak performance from my body, which has resulted in overexertion or injury due to long-term repetitive motion. So, the science and art of Traditional Pilates has been a blessing. Had I known of Pilates earlier in life, I could have prevented such injuries, but I'm thankful now. Today I have more energy; I'm stronger and more protected from eventual injuries compared to most people my age or younger. People perceive me as someone who is strong and without pain, which is relatively true! Living free of physical restrictions and experiencing good energy are extremely important. Joe Pilates wrote: "Physical fitness is the first requisite of happiness. Our interpretation of physical fitness is the attainment and maintenance of a uniformly developed body with a sound mind fully capable of naturally, easily, and satisfactorily performing our many and varied daily tasks with spontaneous zest and pleasure." I am using my personal experience to bring Pilates to more men at a time when most Pilates clients are women.

To my knowledge, most studio owners make some attempt to communicate the benefits of Traditional Pilates to men. One approach is to introduce Pilates at locations where men usually work out or do body conditioning, such as standard gymnasiums. Another good place to introduce Pilates to men is at a martial arts training center or in any other group or individual sports venue involving baseball, basketball, football, skiing, snowboarding, boxing, and so forth. I'm in a fortunate position for many reasons, specifically because I happen to teach classical Pilates to martial artists. There is a lot of good teachers that were also former athletes and involved with martial arts. We are all working to introduce Pilates in realms where athletically disciplined individuals are active. Joe Pilates wanted to bring his method of Contrology directly to public and private educational organizations.

Primary and secondary schools are ideal settings for introducing Pilates because kids learn various sports activities during the course of their education. However, when kids and young adults work toward developing their skills to a high level, demands on the body can cause intense physical stress. Many young athletes can become overexposed to repetitive motion. Some of these young bodies aren't strong enough to endure intense amounts of force and strain that come from repetitive movement patterns. While kids are striving to improve their game, it seems that most parents, coaches, and trainers do not include enough elements of body conditioning in their training, let alone Traditional Pilates. Pilates would provide uniform development with divergent movement patterns and never overexert certain muscle groups with repetitive motion—perfect for the developing athlete.

In my Pilates studio, I have a client who practices the sport of fencing. She's very young, and she trains in fencing six times each week at a very high level. During her initial Pilates lesson, I asked the parents if their daughter was also involved in some form of body conditioning. The answer was no. This is the case with nearly every young athlete. The sport of fencing has asymmetrical movement patterns—as nearly every sport does—that eventually develop certain muscle groups into stronger resources to achieve competitive aims. Naturally stronger muscle groups create significant imbalances that result in more potential for injury and long-term physical damage. This is a major problem that we're finding with children and young adults who are training at high levels in their chosen sport. Since Traditional Pilates creates uniform development of all muscle groups and establishes coordinated movement from core muscles, Pilates should be the foundation of a sound training regimen.

Even in this day and age when Pilates has enjoyed significant commercial appeal worldwide, only a small number of professionals teach Joe Pilates' traditional system of body conditioning. Becoming a qualified teacher takes time, commitment, work, study, discipline--and Pilates training is expensive. As a result, Pilates is missing from the weekly routines of kids and young adult athletes. The problem persists as athletes age, with athletic programs in high schools and universities being primarily invested in the current performance of their athletes. They are not evaluating the future physical needs or the prevention of potentially symptomatic issues later in life.

My background in boxing, sports, mathematics, and chemistry all connect to my understanding and teaching of Traditional Pilates technique. Let's briefly consider these dimensions. Joseph Pilates himself incorporated movements of animals and those of human sports into his system of Contrology. Think of the Arm Series with its Boxing exercise; think of the Fencing exercise. These exercises naturally have similar movement, placement, and carriage. Having knowledge and experience in boxing, I understand that throwing a punch must originate from the core muscles to create the most power. Yet, there's more. Anatomically, there is a musculoskeletal chain starting from the heels, which goes through the hips, Powerhouse, upper back, shoulder, elbow, and down into the glove. Boxing becomes more skillful, powerful, and energy efficient by practicing Joe Pilates' system of Contrology.

One of the most important aspects of any sport is the efficiency of energy consumption. An ineffective moving body uses a lot of energy, meaning that it will get tired fast. A well-trained body, with the right mental conditioning, will use less energy to produce physical activity than an untrained one. When the body is low on energy, skill, technique, and mental strategy suffer. In a well-balanced match, the winner is usually the person whose energy can be sustained through time. Just think of a tennis player or marathon runner. Their expenditure of energy is enormous. As a result, when athletes begin to fatigue, their alignment decreases; their technique becomes inconsistent; more imbalances begin to emerge; and they begin to consume even more energy to reestablish dynamic homeostasis. In Contrology, precision of movement, breathing, stretch, and strength all combine into heightened levels of coordination with efficient use of energy. Thus, we see the useful application of Traditional Pilates in sports. Finally, the study of chemistry and, specifically, biochemistry facilitates my understanding of brain-body connections. All movement requires coordination between neuroelectrical impulses, chemical interaction, muscle activation, and eventually body movement with simultaneous mental awareness and guidance. Chemistry is integral to how the body moves. I teach Pilates through knowledge of these subjects while preserving Joe Pilates' work.

Switching gears, let's think about ways to potentially increase the male clientele in Traditional Pilates studios, as well as encouraging men to become professional Pilates teachers. In Joe Pilates' original studio during the 1920s—1930s, most of his students were male. Over a period of years, however, most Pilates clients and teachers became women. The primary reason was that dancers discovered the value of Joe Pilates' system of Contrology, and most dancers are female. Dancers understood that Joe Pilates' method could help sustain strength, flexibility, alignment, agility, uniform development, balance, responsiveness and physical control, as well as overall health and vitality, naturally extending their careers in dance. Non-dancers valued Pilates for all the reasons described above, yet also for daily poise, posture, and presence. With all these qualities combined, there's a sense in which Pilates sustains youthfulness, both physically and mentally.

We can help various education and fitness professionals understand that Pilates is a foundational system of body conditioning that can be applied to all sports. Joe Pilates studied ancient Greek forms of exercising the body as well as the ancient Chinese form of movement Cong Fu. He trained in wrestling, boxing, and self-defense. These sports are generally practiced by boys, young men, and men of all ages. So the Pilates Method is absolutely applicable to all males to help them become stronger, achieve greater performance, and help prevent injuries. In addition to communicating with education and fitness professionals, it's beneficial for Pilates instructors to teach classes at different locations, giving lectures and demonstrations.

Around the time men reach age 30, they start having repetitive motion symptoms and injuries. Even when men play sports, or work out at the gym, they gradually practice a more limited variety of physical movements as time progresses. Compare this age-related tendency to the wide spectrum of daily physical activities that kids and young adults naturally execute without even thinking twice. Repetitive motion stress can happen on a daily basis in the most normal ways. For example, consider crossing your legs in a sitting position, slouching while sitting or standing, or leaning to one side while standing. Any single repetitive movement pattern will soon strain the body and cause symptoms, which will lead to an inability to move easily and responsively.

In some of Joe Pilates' videos from the original studio, he demonstrates very simple movements, such as standing up, rising from the floor from a sitting position, being able to touch your toes, moving across the floor with hands and feet, and practicing Going Up on the High Chair or Wunda Chair. These physical movements require strength, flexibility, control, and range of motion that gradually decrease with age; but with Contrology, they remain possible. It's only when you don't regularly utilize the body with intelligent physical activity that various symptomatic issues begin to compromise overall health and vitality.

Some male clients are average sportsmen, but their range of motion and ability to move has been so reduced that they repeatedly get injured in their movement. It may be golf, tennis, fishing, swimming, basketball, mountain climbing, carrying children or grandchildren, grocery shopping, mowing the lawn, repairing the car, or something they love to do; yet, without Traditional Pilates technique, their abilities slowly deteriorate, not only because of their age. Their physical readiness and responsiveness become more limited without the dynamic complexities of Pilates. When men preserve the resiliency and agility of their bodies, they feel a sense of vitality and improved concentration.

Adults of various ages say, "I must be getting old," when they perceive a gradual decrease in functional strength, flexibility, coordination, balance, concentration, agility, and responsiveness. Even if a man works out in the gym 3-4 times per week, physical and mental limitations can persist. That's because gym exercise equipment and programs are fragmented; they don't comprise an integrated system like Joe Pilates' method of mental and physical conditioning. It is essential to condition the mind and body simultaneously. This combination is central to Traditional Pilates technique. The Method is mentally complex; therefore, it's necessary to apply cognitive discipline to guide muscular control. If our brain slows down, our body will respond inefficiently and ineffectively. Of course, Joe Pilates understood these points. He was devoted to each individual's health and well-being, and he developed the system of Contrology that optimizes our abilities.

When Joe Pilates met a new student, even before introducing himself, he would sometimes ask, "Can you touch your toes?" He wanted to test people from the outset. Approaches like this get the attention of men because they present a direct challenge! Most frequently when men are challenged, they respond by wanting to overcome obstacles, gain knowledge, and master the technique. So, by Joe Pilates' asking a new male client if he can touch his toes, he shows us how to motivate someone. It's a humbling moment if you can't touch your toes, which makes you want to explore the benefits of Pilates and eventually believe in the system. Joe Pilates used that kind of test to implicitly convey to students: Look, this is The Work; this is where you are; and this is what you can gain if you practice Contrology. Our charge as Pilates professionals is precisely that.

About Alessandro:

In 2007, Aessandro Balboni made a career change and attended the Pilates™ Certification Program in New York City. Alessandro trained for 600+ hours—gaining mastery of all the Classical Pilates apparatus. Alessandro maintains his instructor certification with continuing education seminars at Romana's Pilates. In addition to his Pilates training, Alessandro draws on his experience as a boxer and rower, offering a disciplined and quality level of body conditioning.

Epilogue

Men's Misconceptions of The Work

By Peter Fiasca

Voices of Classical Pilates II: Men's Work focuses on men and their connection to Joe Pilates' corrective exercise system, Contrology. According to 1st generation professionals, Joe Pilates created his body conditioning method for men. Yet in today's world, men have misconceptions about the work, which inform their decision whether or not to study it.

Men's Misconceptions of The Work:

- Pilates is a gentle, feminine stretching activity.
- Pilates does not require strong physical effort.
- Pilates does not include traditional gym exercises such as Push-Ups, Sit-Ups, Bicep Curls, Squats, Leg Curls and Calf Raises.
- Pilates does not build strong physical endurance.
- Pilates does not demand strong mental concentration or coordination.
- Pilates does not increase cardiorespiratory rates enough to get a good workout.
- Pilates is for good posture and aesthetic presentation, but it is not physically challenging.

Men don't realize that Traditional Pilates is a strenuous physical fitness regimen. Misconceptions about The Work interfere with their willingness to try it. Only when they see other men vigorously struggling to achieve a strong workout are they motivated to experience The Work for themselves. Thus, there are very few men who choose Pilates training. Once men learn about Joe Pilates, the master trainer and educator himself, they connect with his strength, skill, drive, and discipline as a human being and accomplished professional.

The Original Studio

During the 1920s, students at Joe Pilates' original studio in New York City were primarily men. Over time the male clientele diminished as women grew in number and comprised the majority of students. Teachers, too, were primarily women. Yet Joe Pilates defined many exercises exclusively for men. He was a tough and demanding physical educator and trainer. During his lifetime in New York City, gender roles were more traditional and less divergent than today. Recent research tells us that whether subtle or striking, men and women frequently demonstrate contrasts in their choice of sports, movement intentions, exercise goals, or technical accomplishments. In spite of sex differences, however, the spectrum of our humanity consistently displays pervasive similarities.

Jay Grimes trained with Joe and Clara Pilates in their original New York City studio. He notes how the passage of time can make anything unrecognizable, including Traditional Pilates technique and teaching. During the 1920s and the next few decades, few people embraced physical exercise routines. At that time, most jobs required more physical exertion than those of today's society. No matter what their occupation, Joe Pilates treated all clients like Olympic athletes; he didn't pamper anyone with gentle teaching or saccharine customer service. Neither did Joe Pilates teach students as if they were injured or fragile. When someone had a physical problem, he discussed it once, briefly. This initial evaluation took place before the client's first lesson. In subsequent workouts, periodically Joe Pilates might teach a specific exercise for someone's physical symptom, depending upon its relative importance; he would simply say, "This is for you," instead of discussing details of anatomy, biomechanics, or kinesiology.

Jay Grimes reminds us of extraordinary social and political changes since the 1920s when Joe and Clara opened their studio. Each student was addressed with their proper salutation of Mr., Mrs., Miss or Dr. as an expected professional courtesy. Casual conversation didn't exist—or scarcely existed—between students or between clients and Joe or Clara Pilates. Time in the studio was primarily dedicated to getting a "medical workout" in the corrective exercise system of Contrology. There was a sense of discipline, propriety, professionalism, formality, and respect. The studio was a tough gym requiring a serious work ethic. You practiced Joe Pilates' system and you vigorously moved your body. No anatomical terms were spoken while teaching. Students might practice Contrology for days or weeks before Joe Pilates offered a single verbal correction. Then he might say, "Pull in the gut" or "Long the leg" or "Down the shoulders," or "Use your arm like a baseball bat." Clara would use her index finger to localize attention on a particular muscle or muscle group.

Joe Pilates did not modify his exercises. Instead, periodically he broke down exercises into component parts, providing useful learning opportunities. Joe Pilates never treated someone like an invalid; he never babied anyone. Even though many students had physical weaknesses, he guided them—without verbally addressing weakness—into using the power of their instinctual movement, animalistic energy, and biomechanics. As a result, people developed their innate ability to increase strength, stretch, control, balance, have coordination and mental concentration.

Exercises Specifically for Men

Joe Pilates taught certain exercises to men that he did not teach to women:

- Swakate Series
- Headstands
- High Bridge
- Low Bridge
- High Frog
- Balance Control Front
- Balance Control Back
- Arm Spring Series

Why would Joe Pilates teach certain exercises only to men? The answer most likely lies in cultural norms and gender role socialization. During Pilates' lifetime, conventional definitions of femininity and masculinity were less divergent compared to today's society. In fact, during the early part of the 20th century, body conditioning was considered a male pastime; in some circles, it was even considered medically unsound, socially improper, or unladylike for women to practice a physical exercise regimen in a gym. In striking contrast, during this same era, women played basketball and tennis, competed in figure skating, swimming, baseball as well as track and field events.

The Traditional Work Benefits Men

What benefits would Joe Pilates want men to learn from his corrective exercise system of Contrology? Consider the following:

- Joe Pilates intended to increase men's functional fitness training. Why? Because he understood that most men condition their bodies with nonfunctional exercises. They isolate muscle groups and rely upon the strength of limbs, independent of the Powerhouse.

- Athletic men inconsistently overexert themselves; they are notorious "weekend warriors." Unless they practice a regular system of body conditioning, these strenuous periodic sports put them at higher risk for potential injury.

- Most men want to feel "the burn" and experience weight load from external resistance.

- Most men have limited understanding of how to develop deep core stability by establishing movement from the Powerhouse; it is very challenging for men to distinguish between external weight load resistance and activation of muscles to create internal muscular resistance.

- Men can indeed learn and benefit from the art of control, which defines Contrology. Achieving optimal effort and coordination in Contrology appears less physically strenuous to the untrained observer, even though muscular intensity actually increases. Most men learn body conditioning techniques that exhibit the opposite: more strenuous effort equals the appearance of more intensity.

Allow Men to Work out - Refrain from Overcorrecting

Men have a natural impetus toward moving their bodies and less interest in receiving verbal correction from teachers. Could this tendency source from gender cultural learning and character development noted earlier? Reflecting upon my own experience, I strongly prefer, and benefit from, teachers who essentially coach me while I'm moving. This way, I get an excellent workout; and, second, I learn something new. Romana Kryzanowska never overcorrected students. And she clearly spoke against the problem. She simply suggested, "Pick out the most important part," which means only identify the most valuable correction—periodically—during the lesson. When I trained with Romana, her silence ironically spoke as poignantly as her words. She intentionally used attentive silence as a teaching tool. The benefits are manifold. Attentive silence allows students: (1) time to reflect *during the workout*; (2) time to comprehend specific exercises *during the workout*; (3) time to anticipate upcoming exercises *during the workout*; and (4) time to experience "poetry in motion," as Romana often said.

There is a spectrum of verbal correction ranging from too much to not enough. If teachers inject excessive correction—no matter how valuable—it can lead to mental distraction as well as overuse injuries from repeating certain movements too often. Overcorrection distorts Joe Pilates' traditional system. Addressing this point, Dr. Roberto von Sohsten and Suzanne Diffine write in their essay, "Affairs of the Heart: Pilates and Cardiac Surgery," "Men must be corrected differently. Don't try to fix every movement or every cycle... If you practice [or teach] OCD Pilates with men, you will fail."[1]

Jay Grimes writes in his own essay, "An Open Letter to Pilates Teachers," "Dear Pilates Teacher, you talk too much!"[2] He explains, "You actually cannot teach Pilates. Pilates comes from within. People have to discover it in their own bodies. You must be their guide."[3] Over time and in various contexts, Jay has discussed the value of silence and quiet observation while teaching. Silence gives students space to learn from their own instinctive, animalistic movement, which requires consistent concentration, physical coordination, and good timing as they challenge themselves and make progress.

Traditional teacher Fredrik Prag echoes the call for minimal verbal communication. In his essay, "The Body Says What Words Cannot," Fredrik writes, "Teaching Pilates to men is all about encouraging them to move with strength and coordination; it is not about verbal correction."[4] These points made by Romana, Jay, and Frederick parallel the first paragraph of Cynthia Lochard's essay titled, "Just Do It." Cynthia emphasizes the importance of allowing men to move without overcorrecting them, "To accomplish Pilates at high levels with exact placement, alignment, balance, and line is an extremely difficult feat; this is where many men lose interest in Pilates, unless they have studied gymnastics or martial arts. Most men like vigorous exercise. They like physical work. They like to move. For them, achieving ideal techn ical forms with the aim of perfection in Pilates is secondary, as it should be."[5]

Conditioning the Entire Body

The corrective exercise system of Contrology necessitates continual activation of one's entire body with interesting combinations of placement and movement. Although this fact is obvious, experiencing a workout involving multi-muscle groups and multi-joint combinations creates a complex and dynamic decision matrix in order to achieve the athletic goals of Traditional Pilates technique. In addition, we increase the potential to improve psychophysiological and neuroimmunological resiliency, which, in turn, strengthens and gradually heals site-specific weakness or injury.[6] There is fundamental value in conditioning the entire body with biomechanically correct exercise in contrast to injury-specific physiotherapy manipulation. In certain cases, and at the appropriate time, however, Joe Pilates would indeed address a specific physical weakness or injury after the entire body develops familiarity with his traditional system. This teaching approach could take several weeks, even months, after the first Pilates lesson. Conditioning the entire body is primary. Dr. John Dalcin speaks to this point in his dialogue with Sandy Shimoda, "Corrective Exercise and Chiropractics: Physician Health Thyself." Dr. Dalcin writes:

> In my chiropractic office, patients regularly utilize Pilates apparatus for neuromuscular retraining—what Joe Pilates called corrective exercise—to reduce challenging symptoms and gain strength, flexibility, coordination, and responsiveness. Pilates provides a system for regaining normal-range, spine/hip mobility; vertebral sequencing; and improved carriage of the entire skeleton as people age. Although the age clock cannot be reversed, individuals can certainly gain strength, flexibility, and control of muscle groups associated with The Center. In turn, daily movements and skilled sports are optimized.[7]

Dr. John Dalcin's points illustrate the value of identifying various physical symptoms while conditioning the entire body. Yet men have challenges integrating all muscles in coordination with Powerhouse muscle groups. Due to gender socialization, peer pressure, and physical training practices, men tend to strengthen muscle groups by isolating them. Establishing movement from the Powerhouse core muscles, then directing that energy through our limbs, is a foreign concept for them. Juan Gabriel Ruiz, in his essay "Pilates: A Gift from My Brother," notes this obstacle for men as they begin training; men practice strengthening exercises for arms, legs, back, and abdominals; but these areas of strength are disconnected from Powerhouse muscle groups. As a result, men have difficulty translating isolated strength into developing a more coordinated and responsive body. Juan Gabriel Ruiz states:

> Usually men force too much energy into the limbs to accomplish physical action because they are unaware of how to connect the Powerhouse with the muscles of the upper and lower extremities. In light of this fact, it's often necessary to slow men's movement so they can understand how to optimize their effort. This way, they discover Powerhouse work and properly direct strength to achieve correct action.[8]

Chris Robinson, another remarkably accomplished instructor, makes a similar point in his essay, "Core Connection." Chris confesses, "Coming from an athletic background and not really understanding Pilates technique at the beginning, I remember trying to muscle through everything. Training with Romana really taught me how to move from the center and really develop core strength. That is something most people don't understand: establishing movement from the Powerhouse is a process that takes time, discipline, study, and expertise." Most men don't understand how to first activate their Powerhouse muscles then direct kinetic effort of core muscle groups through their body's peripheral limb movements.

Correcting Men's Misconceptions

Since men have misconceptions about Joe Pilates' corrective exercise method, how can we help correct these erroneous beliefs? Addressing this issue, Tony Balongo writes in his essay, "Rediscovering Pilates":

Most people don't realize that Joe Pilates created his method for normal healthy bodies and athletes. Of course, it's also brilliant for rehabilitation, yet there is a misconception that Pilates is for gentle stretching and elderly people.

This poses a problem when you think of men potentially training in Traditional Pilates. I remember teaching at a studio that had a gymnasium nearby. Men often walked by the Pilates studio, saw the apparatus and practitioners taking lessons, yet they didn't seem to visually connect with The Method's intense physically demanding work. I'm sure they thought, *Oh, that's kind of that weirdo stretchy stuff.* I know the perception because many men have essentially spoken these same words.

Because I value my work and want to spread the benefits of Classical Pilates, I had to figure out a way to draw them in. So I decided to offer a free class for men at 12:00 noon on Fridays. These big guys came there thinking, *I'm really strong. I can bench press 160 kilograms; I can squat with 325 kilograms.* Within minutes, I had them dripping in sweat. I brought them to the Wunda Chair, put one spring on, and encouraged them, "Come on, do a pull-up." I could almost see blood dripping from their foreheads from the exertion. Then I perched on the pedal, started going up and down, you know, lifting my body up almost like a hydraulic elevator with two legs, then one leg; bop, bop, bop. Their egos deflated, they thought, *What the hell?* Their perception changed.[10]

In their dialogue, "Fit Over 50," José Antonio Lopez and Marta Christina Diaz Velasco expand upon Tony Balongo's assertion that Pilates is perceived by the general public as a feminine body conditioning technique:

People who know that I train with Marta inquire, "Why are you doing Pilates?" They ask because in Latin America there's a macho mentality, a male code of behavior embracing strength, force, dominance, and financial success. Symbolically, they all go together. Yet Pilates is advertised and perceived as women's exercise. It is misunderstood as a feminine activity, which is not physically demanding enough for men. Most men believe you have to train muscles with heavy weights and work them to fatigue. But Joe Pilates understood that building too much muscle mass slows down muscle reaction time in sports, boxing and martial arts...He advocated using your own body weight to develop uniform muscular development...Here's my advice to all men: take a good look at the photos of Joe Pilates demonstrating his system of body conditioning. He was a serious German tough guy, a boxer and athlete. He created a strong method of exercise that enhances every aspect of your life.[11]

The Brain/Body Connection

Moving beyond gender-based and marketplace perceptions of Pilates as a feminine activity, Emre Onuk directs our attention to men's mental health as related to Classical Pilates in his essay, "Pilates: The Mind/Body Connection."

> Depression is no less real here [Ankara, Turkey] than in Western countries. Most often, this is especially a problem for men, because admitting feelings of defeat or acknowledging a mental health issue is seen as weak and unmanly. To those men weighed down not only by their guts, but also by stress, fatigue, and feelings of inadequacy and loneliness, Pilates has brought invaluable relief. What makes their lives better is not only the gain in muscle mass and flexibility, but improved motivation, self-confidence, and the trust in the increased capacity of the mind and body. In our courses and events, we have witnessed this time and time again.[12]

In her essay, "How Can Pilates Combat Slouching and Increase Athletic Longevity in Men?" renowned Olympic ice skater Karen Courtland Kelly reinforces Emre's points regarding the importance of mental health. Kelly never focuses on limitations, instead encouraging her male students to maintain a positive attitude:

> Always keep a sense of humor! Use your gifts to bring out the best in each client instead of imposing limitations. Just ask yourself, *How is that person blocked? Is he thinking about something in the wrong way or is he worried about something?* In athletics, focusing on a negative thought blocks the

pathway to the goal...Clients should feel free and enjoy doing The Work, learning it in a way that enables them to process and enjoy it. Reminding a man to keep his sense of humor is critical to the learning process.[13]

Once men discover the intense discipline and beneficial results of Traditional Pilates technique, they are more capable of living healthy, well-balanced dynamic lives. Yet men continue to encounter negative bias and peer pressure, which discourages them from doing The Work, or even trying it. In their dialogue titled, "Stretch, Strength and Control," by Martin Spencker and Amanda Diatta, it is clear that men still have hurdles to overcome:

> When I tell male friends of mine that I'm training in Pilates, they just laugh! They think it's ridiculous; they have only heard about Pilates when their wives do it after pregnancy to regain urinary control. They have no idea that a tough, strong, intelligent German boxer and inventor named Joe Pilates developed the work for men...These men don't know that Joe Pilates developed a much better system.[14]

Motivating Men: Two Strong Role Models

As times gradually change, so do men's misconceptions about The Work. Today many male professional athletes, college athletes, and recreational athletes benefit from Joe Pilates' vigorous corrective exercise system. In their dialogue, "Growing Up with Pilates," Kathi Ross-Nash and Zak Ross-Nash vividly discuss the integrated system. Zak identifies several benefits of The Work:

> The coaches and players on my team have begun to shift their focus from building as much bulk as possible to developing a combination of strength, flexibility, and speed. To that end, my teammates have experimented with different kinds of body conditioning techniques. Some tried yoga; others, like me, study Pilates. As a result, drastic improvements have been made. We've gone from a sub-500 record to 8-1, among the top 25 football teams in the country. This is awesome. I've shown my friends the science and art of traditional Pilates. They realize that it's actually difficult to practice The Work the

> right way, but my friends keep coming back. Why? Because they get a great workout, and it keeps them playing football.[15]

Zak Ross-Nash is an exemplary role model for the next generation of men who take body conditioning seriously and intelligently, applying their knowledge to the demands of high level sports. As more men realize the value of Joe Pilates' system, they will follow Zak's example. Yet each man will find his own way—within Joe Pilates' system—of developing optimal strength, improving coordination, and increasing overall physical responsiveness for daily movement, recreational activities, and professional sports.

In their dialogue, "Rehabilitation, Resilience, and Vitality," Erik Fridley and Kerry De Vivo discuss how the traditional work helped Erik heal from a sports-related injury. An avid rugby player, Erik is another exemplary role model of the next generation of men who approach body conditioning seriously and intelligently:

> I had herniated discs in my back that eventually required surgery. In addition, I had a rugby injury, a strained right quadriceps, which was the result of a singular event. I must have pulled this muscle because it was extremely tight. That's when Kerry introduced me to Pilates. Neither chiropractic nor physical therapy treatments were effective. Yet when I started Pilates, the pain relief was almost immediate.[16]

Erik has continued to study and train in Pilates, eventually transitioning from rugby to sailboat racing, which is also physically demanding, albeit in different ways from rugby. Erik describes his experience and the benefits of Pilates:

> During this time, there were two big changes in my life: the transition away from rugby and an increased commitment to sailing, which included local and international competitions. In sailing, my biggest improvement was balance. It was a powerful change for me to engage my entire body; sailboats constantly move through linear motion (heave, sway, surge) and rotation (pitch, roll, yaw), tilting, turning, and tipping while the crew works in every position. Pilates enabled me to move more quickly on the sailboat. I developed more agility,

stamina, and strength, climbing the mast without a rope, as if it were a coconut tree![17]

Erik and Zak are remarkable practitioners of the Traditional Pilates system. They don't have misconceptions of The Work. They know that Pilates requires intense strength, adaptability, and intelligence. Their work has surely motivated other men to study Joe Pilates' corrective exercise system. Of course, each man in *Voices of Classical Pilates II: Men's Work* is outstanding. And the women professionals in this collection are among the most highly respected and accomplished. It has been an honor to collaborate with these world-class teachers who are all devoted to preserving the tradition of Joe Pilates.

About Peter:

Peter's unique perspective comes from years of experience as a Romana Kryzanowska certified Pilates instructor. His many years of study, and long-term teacher training experience, culminate into intriguing, spirited and fun educational events! Peter's devotion with Pilates began in 1988, when he took his first class at Wee-Tai Hom's studio in New York City. As his passion grew, Peter pursued teacher training at Drago's Gym, receiving certification in 1998 from famed master teacher Romana Kryzanowska. Over time, Peter honed his knowledge and teaching with regular lessons from Romana, as well as from master trainers Jay Grimes, Kathy Grant, and other distinguished, traditional instructors. Peter continues to study and dedicate himself to preservation of Joe Pilates' traditional system of corrective exercise. Peter helps educate the public about traditional Pilates technique by sustaining the worldwide www.ClassicalPilates.net instructor directory.

Producer and director of the award-winning *Classical Pilates Technique* series of six DVDs (2002-2006) and author of the critically reviewed companion book, *Discovering Pure Classical Pilates* (2008), he has been a frequent guest instructor at training centers throughout the U.S., Europe and South America. Peter's book was translated into Spanish language and titled *Descubriendo el Pilates Clásico* (2010). During 2013 he released a book, *Voices of Classical Pilates*, which is an extraordinary collection of essays written by 28 well-respected professional Classical Pilates teachers. Peter appeared in Romana Kryzanowska's first commercial DVD project, demonstrating the Pilates Mat workout, as well as the DVD *Pilates Revealed*, with master teacher Jay Grimes. During 2017 Peter released *Voices of Classical Pilates II: Men's Work*, which is a unique collection of essays and dialogues by 30 professional Classical Pilates teachers and students.

REFERENCES

[1] Von Sohsten Roberto, M.D., "Affairs of the Heart: Pilates and Cardiac Surgery." Voices of Classical Pilates II: Men's Work. Editors: Bergesen, Amy; Diffine, Suzanne; Fiasca, Peter. 2017.

[2] Grimes, Jay. "An Open Letter to Pilates Teachers." Voices of Classical Pilates II: Men's Work. Editors: Bergesen, Amy; Diffine, Suzanne; Fiasca, Peter. 2017.

[3] Grimes, Jay. "An Open Letter to Pilates Teachers." Voices of Classical Pilates II: Men's Work. Editors: Bergesen, Amy; Diffine, Suzanne; Fiasca, Peter. 2017.

[4] Prag, Fredrik. "The Body Says What Words Cannot." Voices of Classical Pilates II: Men's Work. Editors: Bergesen, Amy; Diffine, Suzanne; Fiasca, Peter. 2017.

[5] Lochard, Cynthia. "Just Do It." Voices of Classical Pilates II: Men's Work. Editors: Bergesen, Amy; Diffine, Suzanne; Fiasca, Peter. 2017.

[6] Fiasca, Peter. "Authentic Pilates and Psychoneuroimmunology." Voices of Classical Pilates, 2013.

[7] Dalcin, John and Shimoda, Sandy. "Physician Health Thyself: Corrective Exercise and Chiropractics." Voices of Classical Pilates II: Men's Work. Editors: Bergesen, Amy; Diffine, Suzanne; Fiasca, Peter. 2017.

[8] Ruiz, Juan Gabriel. "Pilates: A Gift from My Brother." Voices of Classical Pilates II: Men's Work. Editors: Bergesen, Amy; Diffine, Suzanne; Fiasca, Peter. 2017.

[9] Robinson, Chris. "Core Connection." Voices of Classical Pilates II: Men's Work. Editors: Bergesen, Amy; Diffine, Suzanne; Fiasca, Peter. 2017.

[10] Balongo, Tony. "Re-Discovering Pilates." Voices of Classical Pilates II: Men's Work. Editors: Bergesen, Amy; Diffine, Suzanne; Fiasca, Peter. 2017.

[11] De Velasco, Marta Christina and Lopez, José Antonio. "Pilates Fitness Over 50." Voices of Classical Pilates II: Men's Work. Editors: Bergesen, Amy; Diffine, Suzanne; Fiasca, Peter. 2017.

[12] Onuk, Emre. "Pilates: The Mind/Body Connection." Voices of Classical Pilates II: Men's Work. Editors: Bergesen, Amy; Diffine, Suzanne; Fiasca, Peter. 2017.

[13] Kelly, Karen Courtland. "How Can Pilates Combat Slouching and Increase Athletic Longevity in Men?" Voices of Classical Pilates II: Men's Work. Editors: Bergesen, Amy; Diffine, Suzanne; Fiasca, Peter. 2017.

[14] Diatta, Amanda and Spencker, Martin. "Stretch, Strength and Control." Voices of Classical Pilates II: Men's Work. Editors: Bergesen, Amy; Diffine, Suzanne; Fiasca, Peter. 2017.

[15] Ross-Nash, Kathryn and Ross-Nash, Zak. "Growing Up With Pilates: A Conversation." Voices of Classical Pilates II: Men's Work. Editors: Bergesen, Amy; Diffine,

Suzanne; Fiasca, Peter. 2017.

[16] De Vivo, Kerry and Fridley, Erik. "Rehabilitation and The Role of Resilience." Voices of Classical Pilates II: Men's Work. Editors: Bergesen, Amy; Diffine, Suzanne; Fiasca, Peter. 2017.

[17] De Vivo, Kerry and Fridley, Erik. "Rehabilitation and The Role of Resilience." Voices of Classical Pilates II: Men's Work. Editors: Bergesen, Amy; Diffine, Suzanne; Fiasca, Peter. 2017.

www.ingramcontent.com/pod-product-compliance
Lightning Source LLC
Chambersburg PA
CBHW030243030426
42336CB00009B/223

* 9 7 8 0 9 8 9 3 6 9 3 3 6 *